TEARS AND RAGE

THE NURSING CRISIS IN AMERICA

By Jane Schweitzer, R.N., M.P.A.

Adams-Blake Publishing
Fair Oaks, CA

TEARS AND RAGE
The Nursing Crisis in America

By Jane Schweitzer, R.N., M.P.A.

Published by:

Adams-Blake Publishing
8041 Sierra Street
Fair Oaks, CA 95628
USA

First printing 1995

Printed in the United States of America

ISBN 1-883422-05-1

Library of Congress Catalog Number 95-80226

Dedication

For my husband, Al Canton, my most severe critic and my greatest love. I told you I'd get this book done eventually!

With Gratitude...

To all the nurses I've worked with and known throughout my career: I remember you for your unflagging devotion, good humor, and fine expertise. I salute you in your struggle.

Many, many thanks especially to my longtime friends **JoAnn Watson** and **Joyce Forbes**. I will always appreciate your belief in my abilities as a nurse. Your wonderful support was invaluable, giving me the courage to persevere at times when I faltered.

Acknowledgments

Although my name is the one that is on the cover of this book, there are several other individuals who, because of their talent and dedication, made this book possible. I wish to recognize and thank:

Robin Chandler, Head of the Archives and Special Collections Library and Center for Knowledge Management at the University of California, San Francisco. Robin was very professional, conscientious, courteous, and thorough. She was also one of those rare individuals who had the decency to return my telephone calls!

Ruth Letner, who edited the manuscript and offered tremendous encouragement. Ruth's impartial eye changed *Tears and Rage* from a professional moan to a book with direction and a positive conclusion.

Colleen Nihen, Right Angle Productions, whose talent in graphics and in the elusive language of "computerese" created the wonderful cover for this book. Colleen also formatted the manuscript, changing it from a ho-hum, double-spaced hodgepodge, to a real book!

Helen Sperling, Mother-in-law extraordinaire. I am indeed grateful for Helen's input when requested and for her silence when her advice was not solicited. I truly appreciate her caring and support.

Table of Contents

Anatomy of A Nurse's Pocket

Lunch money, life savers, kelly clamp,
bandage scissors, roll of tape,
pen light, stethoscope, alcohol swabs,
tongue blades, cups, ammonia capsules,
straws, pen, pencil, list of patients,
Band-aids, aspirin, lipstick,
pocket guide of nursing diagnoses,
breath mints, knock 'em dead perfume,
map to happy hour.

—*RN Concepts*

PROLOGUE

This is not a book for the faint of heart. If you are looking for something to make you feel good, you'd better shuffle over to the fiction section of the bookstore. This book is, in many ways, a gripefest. In nursing there's a lot to gripe about as well as a lot of griping.

The purpose here is to lay it on the line. All those whisperings in the locker room, the utility room, and the bathroom are shouted out in the following pages.

Most of what is discussed is not new, but here it is out in the open. This in itself is somewhat of a novelty. It's time to speak loudly and clearly about the problems in a very decent profession. There are no pat resolutions to all our gripes. However, my hope is that through this book we can all realize that our complaints are not unique and we are not alone. We are all in this together, for better or worse, whether we like it or not.

For far too long, nurses have been casting off in individual ships, reluctant to be part of our profession's fleet. Now we are changing our solitary courses to a united one as we realize the power of the fleet. Solidarity among nurses is the result of understanding ourselves, our relationship with administrators, managers, doctors, and each other. Perhaps the strongest catalyst for our coalition is the effect that restructuring has on our relationship with patients. The potential dangers of mediocre care have compelled us, as nurses, to reassert our role as primary caregivers and to reassess our perception of ourselves.

At the same time, it's essential to discuss the changes that nurses face as the workplace shifts from the hospital to the community. It is now our task to work with the entire patient to *prevent* illness. This is a major adjustment. For so long, our focus was directed to the individual who was already ill. We are now moving into a more preparatory phase, which is both challenging and frightening. Just the same, change is here and we are here, so let's see how we can make the new ideas work for our benefit and the benefit of our patients.

Threads of commonalty weave through our lives. The thread that pulls us together can also be the thread that pulls us apart. In nursing, **image** is that thread.

Image is a commanding essence that can empower as well as destroy. It involves not only how we are perceived by others in the medical world—administrators, physicians, coworkers, patients, etc.--but also how we are portrayed to non-medical people in books, newspapers, movies, television and even in songs. **Image** also includes how we regard ourselves, an aspect that is particularly destructive and painful to nurses.

Image, which has brought us to our present state of anger and frustration, can also help us resolve the negatives of our profession and move into a new era of self-awareness and self-confidence. It is up to us to untie the knots in this tangled web of our discontent so that we can find the taut lifeline to our future.

It was an **image** of ourselves as helpers, comforters of the sick and wounded that brought us to nursing. Ours was a noble fantasy that brought out the best in us. We saw ourselves bathed in the positive light of respect and high esteem. We would be thought of in the highest manner—by our superiors, by our peers, and by ourselves.

That **image** was indeed a fantasy. Here is the reality. We struggle in the muck of hospital politics, staggering and stumbling through the swamp of demeaning, destructive relationships with doctors, management and, worst of all, with each other. We are lost in trickle-down waste management, headed for the garbage dump. We must renew ourselves by recycling this waste into something usable. For nurses, this means converting discontent to empowerment.

Through empowerment, we can change our own **image** and that of our profession. The key to empowerment is understanding—who we are, how we got to this point, why we act the way we do. Coalition, hopefully, will be the outcome of understanding.

Before understanding, unity, and improved self-image can be attained, it is necessary to identify the problems, gripe about them, and set about eliminating these negatives. At the same time, we must identify and accentuate the positives.

Turn the page. It's time to heal!

CHAPTER ONE

I'm Mad As Hell... Aren't You?

Bitching 101—You Are Not Alone

I get so sick of the garbage of nursing that sometimes I can hardly stand it. I feel a black cloud of anger following me throughout the day. My jaws ache from clenching my teeth. My lips are frozen in a perpetual smile of resignation as I capitulate to the wishes of doctors and management.

Ironically, I really like my job. I like being a nurse, doing that nursing stuff. However, in my vision of being a nurse, I didn't anticipate being a pawn to someone else's bishop in the chess game currently played by physicians and administrators. The idealism of my youth painted a scenario of my patient and me. Anything extraneous was not part of the immediate picture. Of course, there might be a difficult head nurse, but essentially there were no other interferences.

Many years ago in nursing, medical politics was less intrusive than it is today. It was somewhere off in the background, something that physicians grumbled about among themselves. It wasn't the topic of nursing staff meetings. At physician and administration luncheon meetings, hospital dynamics were played out and, subsequently, were reported in hospital newsletters. However, in the '60s and '70s, hospital finances were not as crunched and dire as they appear to be today. In the days before Medicare DRGs (Diagnosis Related Groups), managed care, CTs and MRIs, medicine was not caught up in a financial hurricane. Most situations (purchases of new equipment, renovations, etc.) were handled with some whining, but there was no air of fiscal calamity. Nurses were not faced with possibly being laid off so that the hospital could make ends meet.

Today, all the backroom tap dancing is up close and personal. Nurses are made aware on a regular basis that our job situation is precarious. Big Brother is watching, and any slip in protocol or attitude is duly noted and held in reserve to be used as the ammunition of justification when those pink slips start flying.

I know I'm not alone in this maddening position. Nurses are a legion of 2.2 million in the United States. While I seethe and simmer on my way to work in California, nurses in Massachusetts, South Carolina, and Pennsylvania have already gotten their daily dose of "layoffs are coming; mandatory overtime is starting." It's 9 a.m. for them and their morale is in the sewer. Soon to follow were the nurses in Illinois, Missouri, Colorado, Montana, and New Mexico. Then it's California's turn. By the time the nurses in Hawaii get to work, the majority of the nurses in this country are angry and frustrated for any number of reasons.

In the past, we were only working double shifts, putting in mandatory overtime, and carrying dangerously high patient loads. Now, we are being laid off in droves so that hospitals can realize profits of XX million dollars. As we are replaced by unlicensed and minimally trained personnel—yet expected to supervise them and assume responsibility for their work—patient care is compromised more than it ever was previously. Scenarios of eight or nine years ago have equally frightening corollaries today. Consider:

1986: New York City. A patient at Montefiore Medical Center nearly died when his trachial breathing tube fell out. Reason: No one on the understaffed night shift heard the respiratory alarm go off.

1988: Louisville. For a time, by astonishing coincidence, none of the city's eleven hospitals could accept critically ill or injured patients. Reason: Available beds in intensive care units couldn't be filled because not enough nurses were on duty.

1992: Sacramento, California. A patient, who has just had abdominal surgery, asks the nurse for her pain medication. The nurse refuses. Reason: She is so overworked, she doesn't have time to stop and get the medication.

1995: California. A patient, who is bleeding post-operatively, calls 911 when she is unable to get a nurse to help her.

There is a countrywide morale crisis among nurses, due to lack of autonomy and respect, as well as salaries that fail to reflect the level of responsibility nurses take on each day. We are forced to do more with less, stretch budgets until the Indian on the nickel is riding the buffalo, and do without updated equipment that would enhance the care of patients as well as make our jobs easier. Worn out by stress and unable to cope, nurses are burning out and dropping out, leaving those few who remain at the bedside even more exhausted and frustrated.

> You know you're stressed out when your idea of a great snack during break is Maalox, Nuprin, and coffee.
>
> — *"Nancy Nurse"*

Even though these complaints affect all members of our profession at one time or another, we nurses often feel isolated in our misery, keeping it to ourselves until it's too late and the pot of resentment is boiling over. However, most of us like our jobs, and when we have an especially good day, it's easy to slide into the reverie that "things aren't as bad as they seem." Denial can be very convenient—and very treacherous.

However, denial can go only so far and cover only so much. The situation for nurses in hospitals is miserable and, at times, desperate. This, then, is the garbage of nursing, the universal irritant, the summation of complaints and injustices felt by nurses throughout the country, but rarely discussed openly, if at all. All these interferences crowd out the purpose of nursing: the care of the patient.

Takin' What They're Givin' 'Cause We're Workin' for a Livin'

While nursing organizations seek to provide pat definitions of our profession, we in the trenches are fighting to maintain our sanity, our pride, and our work ethic. As I was compiling the research for this book, I came away with a rather surprising revelation: nursing is a profession in search of definition. The powers that be in the hallowed halls of national organizations have struggled and continue to struggle to provide a sense of who nurses are and what nurses do. Unhappily, their attempts are vague and range from Florence Nightingale's sweeping view of nursing as "how to put the constitution in such a state that it will have no disease or that it can recover from disease" to the definition of nursing by the American Nurses Association set forth in 1980: "the diagnosis and treatment of human responses to actual or potential health problems." These vague abstractions offer little enlightenment. Who are we? We are individuals who make up a profession that is very oppressed.

Being doormats, being abused, and being treated as though we don't have brains in our heads, gets old. Yet, doormatism, abuse, and stupidity seem to go hand in hand with nursing, just like scratching goes with poison oak. We feel lousy about ourselves, and this poor self-image reflects many miserable years and many unpleasant experiences.

Nurses suffer from a situational stupidity that is based on the idea that doing nothing is better than doing the wrong thing. It's OK to take whatever is dished out, and take it with a smile. We are angels of mercy, happy in our role. We proceed without giving much thought to what we do, we blindly go ahead thinking that what we're doing is right, whether it is or not.

This is the stupidity I am addressing: we accommodate ourselves to situations to our own disadvantage—shortened lunch breaks, working overtime, cutting vacations short. Unwittingly, through sacrifices, we allow unacceptable conditions to continue. By offering to put out today's sparks, nurses fail to see the major fires of the future.

Perhaps the term stupid is too harsh or inappropriate. From a more generous point of view, we might determine that stupid actions stem from one's ignorance of possible harmful consequences to you or your department, or despite knowing the possible results, proceeding anyway. It is the latter that causes trouble. Managers will not need to hire personnel if part time or per diem nurses are willing to work extra hours. Breaks are a legal right, but it's easier to pass them up and do the work than to bear the nasty looks of a beleaguered senior staff nurse. Also, there's always some goody-two-shoes waiting in the wings to seize the moment and make those who stand up for themselves look bad ("Oh, I don't mind giving up my break, I had one three weeks ago."). Worse yet, it is such stupidity that allows nurses to be doormats.

On the road through nursing school and immediately afterward, nurses learned to be doormats. It's the profession's persona: absorb the blame, don't fight back, somehow everything is your fault, so just own it and move on. Nurses try to melt into the background, hoping the controversy will subside soon and the incident will not be reported.

Doormatism is treacherous because it's disguised as cooperation and the reward for such cooperation is relative job security. Doormatism doesn't invite reprimands and it looks good on that marvelous instrument of coercion, the annual performance review (aka the annual report card). After all, what nurse wants to be called on the carpet and told: "You aren't doing things our way." or "Dr. Jones complained that you argued with him about..." God forbid a nurse should show any kind of thinking that might be different or revolutionary (the "R" word!). The maverick nurse is indeed a rare breed, if not an endangered species. Of course, suggesting to a physician that his or her way might not be the best way can be professional suicide. I once mentioned to a surgeon who was struggling with a tiny incision (in an area where the scar would never be seen) that it might be easier to enlarge the incision. He did, a few minutes later, after he had lambasted me for making the suggestion. The nurse who questions or thinks is regarded by superiors as a troublemaker. Initiative that is heralded and, indeed, sought after in the business world is stifled in nursing and marks the beginning of the end for that brave soul who sought to improve a situation. To be a doormat guarantees a decent annual merit review. It insures job security and, theoretically, makes life easier all the way around.

Of course, the doormat nurse gets walked on, especially when dealing with other nurses. When we indebt ourselves to others by asking "Will you take my call?" or "Will you work my Saturday for me?" we set ourselves up for never-ending doormatism. Now, we are obligated to our co-workers, so we can't rock that boat either. Otherwise, those reciprocal favors we have counted on for so long will not be forthcoming. Time and time again, we set ourselves up to be abused and taken advantage of by the people we work with each day.

Nurse abuse is a not new. However, as a term of the '90s, it is being defined and refined with each incident. It's no longer as obvious as a surgeon throwing a syringe across the room with such force that it jams into the wall as if it were a knife hurled into a tree. Unhappily, these situations still exist, although not as often as in the past.

Today we're subjected to a more discreet form of abuse. It's subtle, but perhaps more damaging because it can't be pinned down. How many times have nurses been left feeling rotten by the way something was said? Negative comments ("Why don't you people ever listen?" or "The doctor's time is very valuable; the nurse's time is expendable.") are easy to describe. It's more difficult to deal with an attitude or a tone of voice or a shrug of dismissal. Sarcasm has long been a verbal weapon. However, it, too, is gradually being replaced by the impatient sigh, the drumming fingers, and the rolling eyes.

Here's a surprise: I'm not just talking about the way doctors treat nurses. Abusive also describes the way management treats nurses and the way nurses treat each other. In the struggle to maintain our own sense of ourselves, we all beat each other up (backstabbing becomes a way of life). Every day offers a renewed version of *Rocky*. It's not bloody, but it is nasty.

A part of each of us wants to say, "Abuse is ancient history. It applies to older nurses, the ones who used to give up their seats to doctors. It doesn't apply to the young, hip nurses of today, the ones with college and postgraduate degrees. No way." Wrongo, sweetie! We're all in this together. Good news: our ship is in. Bad news: it's the Titantic! If you haven't seen yourself yet, look harder.

I Look in the Mirror and What Do I See?

Our reflection reveals the essence of our profession. Look beyond the fatigue, into your eyes and you will once again see why you are a nurse: you're caring, kind, and considerate.

> Any nurse who can provide the patient with a sense of hopefulness has the true gift of healing.
>
> —*Patty Wooten, RN*

We are nurses. We are healers. This is the image that brought us to nursing. It is also the image that has been eroded by criticism.

"Criticism," the writer Octavio Paz tells us, is "the acid that dissolves images." Applying this philosophy to nursing, we can see that over the years, as we were inundated by criticism, our initial good intentions and idealistic values vanished. We finally caved in and assumed the negative persona that had been relentlessly heaped upon us. We fought to maintain our pride and self-respect. Our poor self-image, the devil within, eventually came to the surface. Unhappily, we also were, and continue to be, assaulted from without.

Don't Look Now—But More Fun Is on the Way!

The enemies within and without are known and long-standing, and nurses are in serious danger of coming to grips with them. Such a confrontation will not take the world by storm; rather a breeze of discontent is blowing. That is an achievement in itself.

As we start to pull ourselves out of our victim mentality, we're about to be hammered again. This time it's the federal government and health care reform, which is preceded in many areas by managed care. The face of nursing is changing. Look out! Look out! All of this, together with its attendant speculation, has thrown hospitals, insurance companies, and doctors into a panic. It has also changed nursing roles (read: jobs) in hospitals and other areas of traditional nursing. Hoping to offset rising costs, hospitals are relying on fewer nurses and more nursing assistants. As the focus of care appears to be shifting from the patient to the dollar bill, we nurses are trying to make our concerns known at both the state and federal government levels.

We are also looking at other possibilities within the scope of our profession and we are intrigued, albeit somewhat wary, about the future. Nevertheless, it is a new era that allows us to have charge over our perceptions of ourselves and ultimately over our own destinies.

Indeed, the changes forced on us may truly be blessings in disguise. The veterans are forced to take some long-awaited action, and the more career-minded new kids on the block, will get through the muck of the past and go on with a strong, positive stride.

How Did We Get Here from There?

Here is now; there is then. It has taken a long time—over 100 years—for nurses in the United States to get to the boiling point. The breathtaking sail through the preceding paragraphs brought us to just the tip of the iceberg (back to the Titanic again!). It's time to slow our pace so that we can understand what happened to bring us to this precipice of desperation and controversy.

CHAPTER TWO

"Twenty Years Of Schooling And They Put You On The Day Shift"

Emerging from the Battlefields

It has been over a century since Florence Nightingale was crawling around the Crimea, helping soldiers who were dropping like flies and writhing on the ground in the stench and agony of battle. It is an irony of nursing that the greatest strides in the profession were made as a result of wars: Crimean War, Civil War, and World Wars I and II, Korean War, and the Vietnam War. Yet, settings such as these also provided the image that has plagued nursing with its inevitable stereotype: the shadowy caregiver lifting the head of the dying soldier, offering solace in his waning minutes. Florence Nightingale gave us our profession. Unfortunately, she also gave us conflicting images that continue to plague us today.

By the time Ms. Nightingale came upon the scene, nursing was in a pre-Victorian abyss. Women took care of family members in the home. Nursing religious orders faded with the demise of the Roman Catholic Church in England. Institutional care fell into a nether world of criminals, alcoholics, prostitutes, and those who had been previously ill. It was a wretched limbo, to say the very least. Nurses were a shabby lot who were regarded, even by Florence Nightingale, as "those who were too old, too weak, too drunken, too dirty, too stolid, or too bad to do anything else" (Nightingale, [1867]).

Florence Nightingale was a true product of her times. A member of the privileged class, she set her sights on repaying her debt to society by restoring nursing to an honorable and respectable rank. Women were regarded as naturals for a calling that required moral superiority, sensitivity, and warmth. Nurses were women doing "women's work" in a world that regarded women as second-class citizens.

Despite her own aristocratic background, Florence Nightingale regarded nurses as beneath her. Nurses were servants relegated to the dismal trappings of that class: small Spartan rooms, meals with the other servants in the kitchen and long hours. Nursing was a blue collar job done by second-class citizens. The stage was set.

From the Poorhouses

In the United States, the first recognized nurses realized similar struggles. In the early part of the 19th century, when women performed private nursing duties in the home, their assignments were specific: childbirth, terminal illness, etc. The quandary of whether to consider nurses as highly regarded domestics or as professionals was not entertained seriously, so nurses moved easily within the confines of a very social-conscious society. Simultaneously, another type of nursing began to surface in the poorhouses and slums of large cities. The ill in these dire circumstances found comfort among women of their own class, rough and tumble individuals who knew nothing of the niceties of "parlor nursing." More often than not, these nurses were also in various stages of recovery themselves. As in England, the stereotype for American nurses was set in motion.

Before the 1870s, there was no such entity as a trained nurse. Upper class women, horrified by existing hospital conditions, recognized the need for trained nurses and pushed to establish nursing schools. This was done, despite resistance from physicians, who were threatened at the prospect of independent, educated women who might not do as they were told (some things never change!).

However, these upper class women were individuals with a purpose, and they persisted. They were not seeking physician approval to succeed in bringing nursing respectability. Indeed, physicians were bypassed if necessary, as these women sought the assistance of other men of status (bankers, lawyers, etc.), who had more power and authority in raising money to build decent hospitals and establish desperately needed nursing schools.

The three nursing schools established in the United States by 1873 multiplied to 432 by 1900 and 1,192 by 1910. These schools were the early training grounds for middle class women who wished to work outside the home. Nursing education was achieved in programs closely associated with and developed by hospitals. These diploma programs took three years to complete and, in most cases, included boarding at the school. There were no college courses included in the

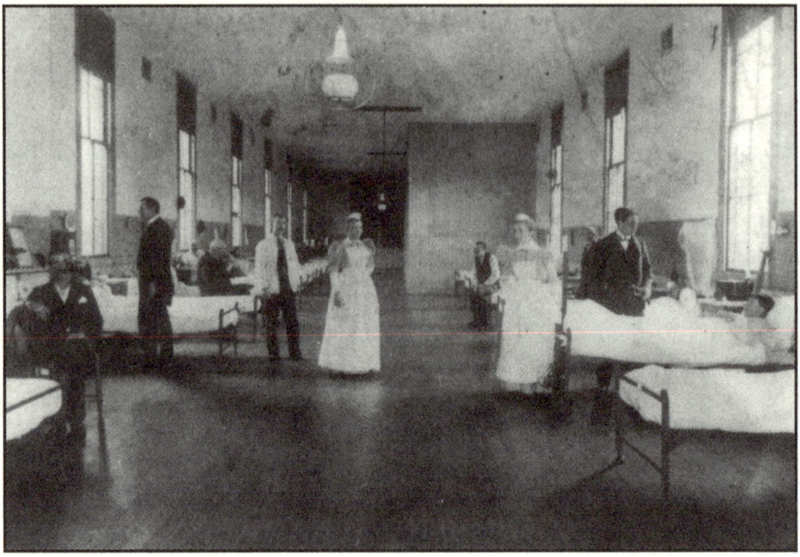

Nurses on the ward at San Francisco General Hospital c. 1890. (Courtesy UCSF archives.)

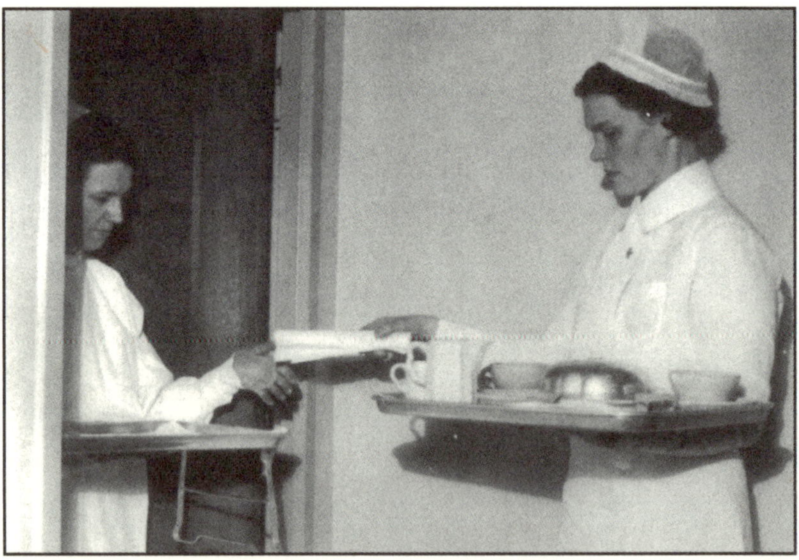

Nurses serving meals at San Francisco General Hospital c. 1940. (Courtesy UCSF archives.)

curriculum. Rather, this was an in-depth program for women with no further designs on education.

Nursing continued its appeal in a steady, positive climb. Despite the nearly 70,000 military nurses who were commissioned after World War II, the war created a nursing shortage. Nurses found conditions and pay in the military superior to civilian nursing positions. In 1946, civilian staff nurses were earning less money than typists and seamstresses. This nursing shortage eventually led to the development of one year programs that produced licensed practical nurses (LPN) or licensed vocational nurses (LVN).

While the first university-based nursing program was established in 1909 at the University of Minnesota, it wasn't until the mid-1960s that Bachelor of Science degrees in nursing were regarded as the norm. In addition, two-year registered nurse programs, available through junior colleges, conferred Associate in Arts degrees.

By the 1960s, the educational spectrum was wide open. Programs of two, three, and four years were available to those wishing to be registered nurses. Very little, if any, recruiting was necessary. Nursing schools were turning away hordes of applicants, filling available slots effortlessly. The best and the brightest were accepted on the strength of banner grades and essays that set forth the reasons they chose a career in nursing.

Gradually, men began filtering into the profession. The Vietnam War produced corpsmen who had significant medical skills. These men did not intend to start all over when they returned home from the war. Nursing offered an opportunity to step into a career, using the expertise they already possessed, without extensive years of education and training.

Although they comprise only 6.2% of the 2.2 million nurses in the United States, men are recruited by the profession. Yet, nursing remains a woman's profession, with all attending negative stereotypes very much intact.

"I Want to Be a Nurse Because..."

Pick a reason, any reason:

> "I want to save the world."
> "I need a meal ticket."
> "Blood doesn't bother me."
> "I like people."
> "I look good in white."
> "It seemed like a good idea at the time."

The young and idealistic are inevitably caught up in the desire to help people. Theirs is the mental utopia presented in Hollywoodesque fashion: the benevolent shade caressing the forehead of a stricken wreck of humanity. They envision a world where, as nurses, they will make a difference, where they can offer comfort and solace to the ill and their families, where they can teach what they know to students and patients alike. This is the way young nurses want their world to be and, in some respects, this is the way their (and our) world ought to be.

Unfortunately, this is not always reality. The idealists are the nurses who are the most frequently disappointed and disillusioned by their choice. They are the ones most likely to drop out and seek to have their idealism fulfilled through other means.

The more practical individuals opt for nursing as a guaranteed meal ticket. Nurses can travel and get a job with certainty wherever they happen to light, whether it's Cicely, Alaska or Pitchfork, North Dakota. New options in nursing offer varied careers (consulting, traveling nurses, nurse practitioner) throughout the country and the world. This is job security at its best: nobody's left on base!

The development of medical technology has opened new areas for nursing practice. The specialties have become increasingly refined. A surgical nurse can become part of the heart team, working specifically on open heart surgeries. Ambulatory surgery centers are fast-paced and handle short, quick cases for those who like speed and variety (and who aren't afraid to rely on in-line skates!). As physicians open their own operating room facilities, they recruit nurses to work for them in their specialties: ear, nose and throat surgery; plastic surgery; ophthalmic surgery. There are pediatric specialists, coronary care, and surgical intensive care nurses. Home health care has spawned "ostomy" nurses who care for and teach those with colostomies, iliostomies, tracheostomies, etc.

Nursing offers a veritable menu of options, so that anyone can find a niche (see chapter 10 for an extensive discussion of this subject). Should boredom or burnout set in, nurses can shop around and seek educational refresher courses in other areas. Medical insurance companies regularly seek nurses for utilization review and management posts. Another market that has opened up in recent years is the "Dial-a-Nurse" concept. Through an advertised telephone number, people from around the country solicit referrals and advice. This lets nurses get off their feet, work flexible hours, or earn some extra money.

While nursing has offered the security of a "meal ticket," the profession has never been known to command phenomenal salaries. Money has never been a strong incentive to enter nursing. However, the situation is improving. It's still not great, but there's hope! Many of the specialties command higher salaries than those of a generic nurse. Some hospitals have initiated the step system, whereby salaries reflect specialty certification and advanced educational efforts. In-house registries allow employees to work additional shifts for pay above shift differentials and overtime salaries. Nevertheless, salaries are not adequate compensation for the grueling work that is required of nurses. The hours, too, are long with shift rotations, weekend, and holiday work. Vacations are given grudgingly, with guilt frequently attached to the approval. Some specialties require emergency call, which may demand from 24 to 48 hours of nonstop work.

> A nurse should be kind, speak gently, love much, and laugh often.
>
> —*L. Seaman*

The idea of professionalism is appealing. "Nurses do what I could never do" is a common refrain. We are patient advocates, trusted and revered. However, at times professionalism is compromised and ceases to be a reality, let alone a guiding force. Since long-established practices and ideas do not willingly fade, even today we nurses frequently find ourselves caught in a web of damaging relationships—nurse/media, nurse/nurse, nurse/doctor, nurse/management—that defy cracking with a jackhammer.

CHAPTER THREE

Lights...Camera...Action: Media Magic

That's Entertainment!

Nursing as a profession is as mysterious as it is misunderstood by the general public. The battle of image that occurs outside our profession also perpetuates and fosters negative images of nurses: bimbos, easy sexual conquests, gold diggers looking for rich doctors to marry, bitches with diligent agendas to destroy beleaguered patients, starry-eyed graduate nurses, and losers who have nowhere else to go. The media takes on nursing with a vengeance. Movies, books, television, the evening news, and even political cartoons have a hand in creating a disparaging concept of nurses. Who could possibly be better suited to tell the world how nurses function, what makes nurses tick than the reliable newscaster, reeking of pompous sincerity?

What a relief it is to have Madison Avenue, Hollywood, and the deities of the six o'clock news setting the world straight on nurses!

You Ought to Be in Pictures...

Hollywood made us larger than life (Oh, joy! Oh, rapture!). Jennifer Jones looked out at us in black and white, dewy and doe-eyed, excruciatingly dedicated in *For Whom the Bell Tolls.*

The past twenty to thirty years has been dismal for the Hollywoodization of nurses who have been portrayed as self-deprecating subordinates of limited competence in a profession that is predominantly feminine. Nurses suffer degrading stereotypes, such as the sexual mascot or the officious drill sergeant bitch. The movie moguls have made fleeting attempts to make us look good, but the real money is in presenting fiends like Nurse Ratchit in *One Flew Over the Cuckoo's Nest* or sexpots like "Hot Lips" Houlihan in *M*A*S*H.* The viewing public loves to have a target to shoot at and nurses have filled the bill all too often.

Reluctantly, movie titans sometimes portray nurses in admirable, sympathetic roles in films like *The Nun's Story* and *The Elephant Man.* Unfortunately, films of this complimentary genre are too few.

Our image on the silver screen has been mirrored on television as well. While programs like *The Nurses* and *Nightingales* were insulting and degrading, *China Beach* and some episodes of the *M*A*S*H* series were sensitive and appropriate, revealing some awareness for what nurses really do, albeit in a military, wartime setting.

There is definitely a lack of decent films and programs that might accurately reflect the daily lot of nurses. A public television special aired in the fall of 1993 was a happy exception. This cinema verité presentation dealt with intensive care and emergency room nurses, nurse anesthetists, etc. It focused on nursing in an objective, truthful manner and made one proud to be part of such a commendable profession. Still, television remains ambiguous in its portrayal of nurses. On one hand, the producer of *Nightingales*, Aaron Spelling, has created a series, *University Hospital*, that is just as insulting to nurses as *Nightingales.* Yet another program features nurses as the ones who run the emergency department capably and efficiently.

However, it is the invisibility of nurses in the news media that strikes the most painful chord. Rarely interviewed as experts, nurses are cast in the anonymous role of backdrop while a physician nods his (occasionally her) head thoughtfully.

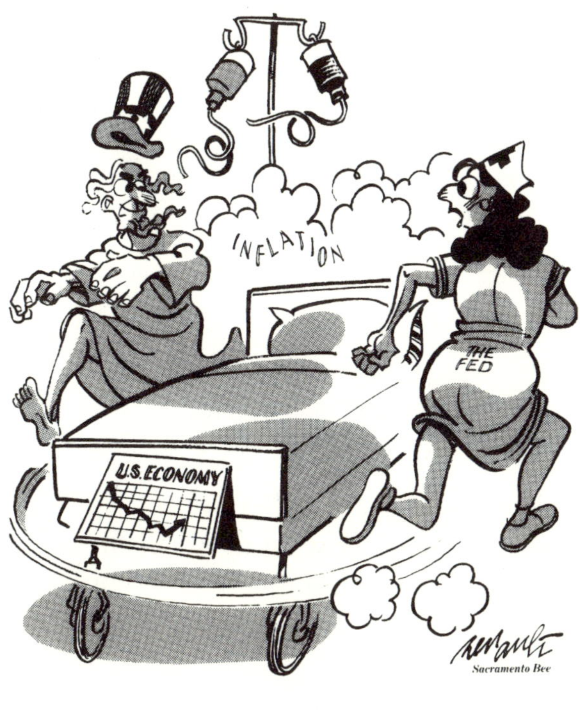

"I'm glad you're feeling better but you mustn't get overheated!"

Political cartoons make their point by presenting uncomplimentary caricatures of their subjects. (Courtesy Dennis Renault, *Sacramento Bee*, 1994.)

Relying solely on physicians as founts of uncontested knowledge and resource is both annoying and ironic since it is nurses who, totally involved in patient care, can give up-to-the-minute assessments. It is nurses who provide doctors with the information that they so knowingly provide on the evening news. It would be gratifying to see a nurse regarded in a positive light, such as a spokesperson on a newscast rather than as a malcontent on a picket line who theoretically jeopardizes the lives of patients or as a misguided angel of mercy responsible for the systematic deaths of those in unrelenting pain.

The visuals presented by the media also affect those who are considering nursing as a career. This, of course, depends on what movie or television program is popular, at the time. *Dr. Kildare, Ben Casey* and even *St. Elsewhere* were unwitting little recruitment vignettes. Although nurses were not portrayed as rocket scientists, they were, nevertheless, individuals to be admired and emulated. While these portrayals tapped shallow reservoirs, they projected somewhat positive visual images of nurses and got people thinking about the possibilities of nursing as a profession.

Bill Moyers' PBS special, *Healing and the Mind,* set forth a fine portrayal of nurses as caring, dedicated, and knowledgeable professionals. The camera captured thc cssence of nursing as it studied extensively the daily activities of two nurses who worked in the special care nursery of a Texas hospital. However, even Moyers capitulated to the thinking that what was being described went beyond nursing, that this was, in fact, *medicine.* The idea that anything complex and holistic might be totally within the parameters of nursing seems hard to grasp. Nursing is supposed to be basic, simple hand-holding. Anything that surpasses these attributes must be *medicine.*

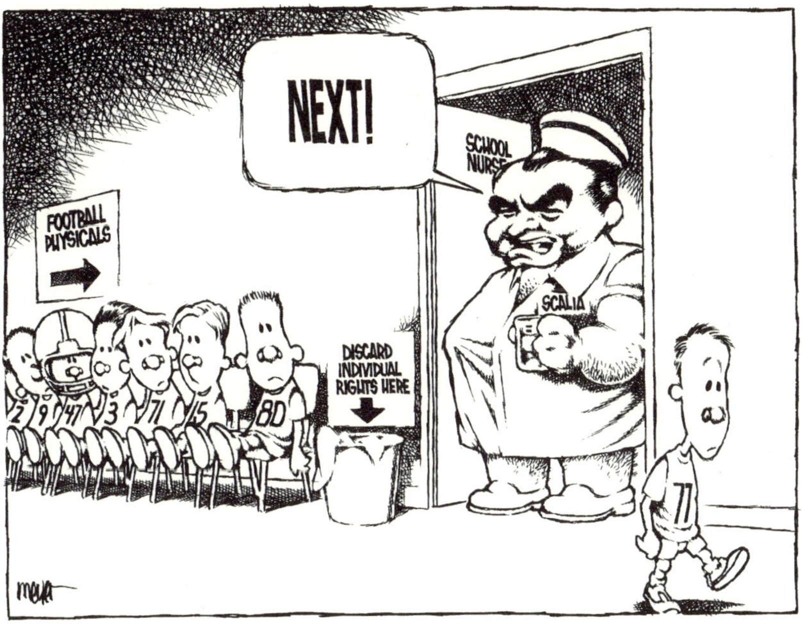

(Courtesy Tom Meyer, *San Francisco Chronicle*, 1995.)

More recently, television programs like *ER* and *Chicago Hope* offer more realistic views of hospital work and the role of nurses. These current shows are hard-hitting and don't waste time being cute. Doctors and nurses are shown working together as a team. The work is hard and the viewer comes away with a better understanding of how tough it is to be in medicine.

Yet, despite the effort to be more accurate in their portrayals of nurses, television inaccuracies still contribute to a negative nursing image. A recent survey conducted by the American Nurses Association showed that 85.2% of those responding thought inaccurate depictions of nurses in television dramas and sitcoms hurt nursing, and 71.4% thought such portrayals hindered recruitment into the profession (*The American Nurse,* March 1995, p. 31).

Books, Books, Books

The written word and many films taken from books are also far from flattering toward nurses. *One Flew Over the Cuckoo's Nest* with the nasty, yet memorable Nurse Ratchit is such an example.

Well-known author, Faye Kellerman, writes compelling mysteries that are suspenseful and timely. In her book, *Grievous Sin*, the characters run the gamut of professional sickies, such as the male RN in a nursing home who siphons pocket change from the patients. This same RN, capitulating to blackmail, allows a psychotic LVN to use his nursing license. Another RN who works in a hospital nursery kidnaps a baby and kills a nursing trainee. The nurses who are not mentally compromised are portrayed as overworked, burnt-out martyrs who take what's dished out rather than making waves.

Kellerman tries to even matters by addressing pertinent issues like floating, layoffs, and shortstaffing. However, these are mentioned in passing. The strongest words against being shortstaffed, uttered by a nurse who is a true victim and martyr, sound like bitter clichés: "We often have to do double or triple our load because some cheapskate administrator would rather have new office furniture than hire needed staff" (*Grievous Sin*, p. 270).

Margaret Mitchell's *Gone with the Wind* gave us Scarlett O'Hara and Melanie Wilkes offering their limited nursing skills for the cause of the Confederacy. They were southern genteel women who slipped into their designated nursing roles as was expected. As the remnants of the Confederate army lay about the outer reaches of the Atlanta hospital, Ms. Mitchell tantalized her readers with vivid descriptions of the appalling medical inadequacies created by the war. The story's heroines were desperately bandaging wounds, offering water and comfort and assisting in gruesome amputations. It was this final task that caused Miss Scarlett to throw up her hands in repulsion and stalk back to Tara in a snit!

Even historical books portray nursing as uniquely women's work. While their husbands are at the battlefront cheering the lads, the Duchess of Windsor, Tsarina Alexandra (the last empress of Russia) and her daughters are depicted in their predictable and prescribed roles devotedly rolling and sorting bandages and tending to the wounded. These well-known women who performed stereotypical duties were regarded as sterling examples for their gender.

"Song Sung Blues"

It was bound to happen. But it was a shock nevertheless to realize that negative images of nurses exist even in the lyrics of songs. Granted, *Desolation Row* appeals to a select audience, but that doesn't change the image.

Bob Dylan, that notable balladeer who gave us *Blowin' in the Wind, The Times They are A'Changin'* and *Lay Lady Lay* wrote many intriguing and complex songs. Given his sensitivity, it is disappointing to find the following lines in *Desolation Row*:

> Now his nurse, some local loser
> She's in charge of the cyanide hole
> And she also keeps the cards that read
> "Have Mercy on His Soul"

I can't wait to have her take care of me. What have you done to us, Bob?!

CHAPTER FOUR

Nursing Politics

The Backstabbers: Why We Don't Get Along

Several years ago, while concluding an interview for a position as an operating room staff nurse in a local hospital, the department manager looked at me and warned, "This is a very catty OR."

Rather than being taken aback, I smiled at the honesty. "All ORs are catty," I replied.

"Yeah, but this one's worse than most."

Backstabbing is an integral part of nursing. It is a means of survival. Medicine is a world of tension, where a medication error can be fatal, a patient may take a turn for the worse with no warning whatsoever, or a new mother may begin hemorrhaging suddenly. In such a world where little gratitude is expressed and criticism and negativity are the rule rather than the exception, backstabbing offers a degree of compensation. Women are not confrontational by nature. It's easier for them to get anger and aggressions out by indirectly complaining about an offending party instead of facing the foe head-on. Not only does one get rid of a gnawing irritation by avoiding a face-to-face discussion, but one also avoids the risk of further assault. This allows one to save face and to massage a wounded ego.

Those who suffer from a poor self-image are probably the worst offenders. They constantly try to feel better about themselves at the expense of colleagues, God, country, and mother. Complaints that start out as professional gripes often end up as personal attacks.

"What do you expect from her, she's so self-centered. If she wasn't so busy talking about herself, she might remember to pull those instruments and you wouldn't spend the entire case running."

"Of course, Joseph didn't report that the microscope was broken. He's out there in Josephland."

"Jean is so perfect. I wonder what it's like to be so marvelous."

"Did Paul come here to work or to socialize?"

"It was great! I finally got her off her butt and had her running all morning."

The lounge becomes the site of major group therapy sessions where tears are cried and plummeting self-respect is rescued. Apart from the sense of satisfaction it provides, another upside of backstabbing is that it also promotes group support. This is especially true when the target is a universally disliked colleague or doctor. As woes are aired, sympathetic listeners eagerly await their moment to jump in with their own tales of unpleasantness with the individual currently on the verbal rack. War stories fly back and forth and the negatively charged atmosphere elicits a strange camaraderie among those similarly wronged.

If we nurses are tough on each other, we are much tougher on physicians (no surprise here). For the most part, nurses are on an equal footing with each other. However, the "equal" footing between doctors and nurses is as tenuous as Los Angeles during an earthquake.

Nurses are treated like sponges—we are there to soak up the blame and the criticism. Once, while working an on-call shift on a Sunday, a surgeon berated me for not answering the telephone promptly. I explained that we were repairing a fractured hip on an elderly patient and with all the equipment buzzing and roaring and the general din in the room, I was unable to hear the phone ring. "You should have been looking at the phone to see if the light was blinking," he charged. Silly me! If I'm unable to hear the phone ring, logic dictates that, of course, I should keep my eyes glued to the phone on the chance it might ring. Never mind the patient or the demands of the current situation.

On another occasion, an elderly patient was brought to surgery for a cardiovascular procedure that involved the lower part of the body. Because of health problems, the anesthesiologist opted to give a spinal anesthetic rather than a general anesthetic. In preparation for this, the patient was given medication for relaxation.

"We want you to sit up now and face the nurse," the patient was instructed.

With some difficulty, she managed to sit. But, sleepy from the medication and quite a bit overweight, the patient swayed and slumped intermittently as she drifted in and out of her narcotically induced stupor. Not only was the patient a moving target, but also degenerative changes in her spine had closed normally opened intervertebral spaces where the spinal anesthetic was to be introduced. It was an awkward situation since the patient was very difficult to hold.

"Hold her still," the doctor barked. "Don't let her move!"

"She's moving, for chrissakes! Will you just hold her?!"

The nurse pointed out that the effects of the medication contributed to the difficulties. This was not well received. After considerable time and fumbling, the anesthesiologist gave up and the patient was laid down on the table.

"I could have gotten the spinal in if you had done your job," the anesthesiologist said.

"I will not accept the blame for your failure. You need to accept responsibility for your own garbage and not blame everyone else," countered the nurse.

The doctor's response was to have the nurse removed from the room. This provided ample fodder for locker room discussion, especially since the scrub nurse was also in the room at the time and couldn't wait to take up the cause on behalf of her co-worker

Even benign disagreements on a personal level can create problems. A discussion between a doctor and a floor nurse about the nurse's home state on the East Coast was cause for a dispute when the doctor made a disparaging, unfounded comment, and the nurse rose to the defense of her home.

"She is very argumentative," the doctor later complained to the senior staff nurse.

"Don't argue with the doctors," the nurse was subsequently admonished. "We can't afford to lose the business."

This provided a double whammy: verbal target practice on the physician ("He's a jerk, anyway.") and the senior staff nurse ("Don't you love how the staff has management support around here?").

Under such circumstances, it is easy to understand backstabbing. It's a means of fighting back. It's a way of saying "If so-and-so is so stupid or can act like such a fool and I don't act that way, I must be OK." By putting others down, we delude ourselves into thinking that we have resurrected our own credibility and pride. It's not pretty, but it works.

And the Winner Is...

Competition is healthy, we are told as children. It brings out the winning spirit, the do-or-die effort. These assertions are valid in baseball, Scrabble, and spelling bees. A competitive spirit, however, produces very different consequences in nursing.

For nurses, competition is not a tool for fine-tuning skills and abilities, rather it is a weapon that is used to insure success, regardless of the effect on one's peers. Competition is borne out of jealousy, poor self-esteem and the desperate need for recognition and respect. Whereas most businesses strive to achieve a spirit of cooperation among employees, nursing instills the need to compete. We don't compete to win; we compete to stay alive.

This competition of negativity is one of the great weapons of management and administrators. In his article, "Professional Jealousy—the No-Win Factor" (*Revolution–The Journal of Nurse Empowerment*, Winter 1994), writer Harold Stearley points out that "By keeping nurses divided [read: competing] between units, shifts, new-hires, and experienced staff; associate, diploma, bachelor degree credentials; and favorites and outcasts, managers create an impotent, fractionated workforce." Stearley continues, "...when infighting and backbiting are the rule, administration has less to worry about because nurses who are divided don't unite to fight for better working conditions." The result is that all our negative images are reinforced as we struggle with an impotence generated not only by our own actions, but also by the methods employed by management and administration. For nurses in the trenches, competition provides no winners.

The Nurse Manager: Devil with the Blue Dress On

Nurse managers are an interesting breed. Since they usually come up through the ranks, they are not strangers to the plight of staff nurses. They've been there before, right? They've suffered the consequences of understaffing. They know the desperate feeling of being overworked, of caring for 20 patients at a crack, of doing case after case with no coffee break or lunch in sight. When they take over the reins of our department or unit, there is a sense of satisfaction that one of us has made into the hallowed halls of management. We smile. We know things will get done, long-awaited goals will be accomplished, and grievances will be corrected. The preceding ogre is gone and hope is our ally again. We know our leader is worthy of us and any fleeting doubts are ushered to the back of our minds as we launch into a mythical probationary period. We don't expect failure.

The initial period is one of great activity. Very often, there are overt signs of positive change. Files are reorganized, ancient equipment is deployed to the Smithsonian, problem employees are gently counseled, and innovative ideas are tested and explored. During this time, morale is high and even the most jaded among us grunts reluctant approval.

Then it happens. There is a shift. It's so subtle, it's almost elusive. You can't put your finger on it, but it happens. Was it when the nurse manager stopped wearing a uniform or scrub clothes? Did it occur with the donning of the crisp, starched lab coat emblazoned with the manager's name? Our advocate is slowly slipping away to the other side, to become one of "them." Somewhere along the line, our manager stopped being a nurse and became a member of the administration. Phrases like "in the black," "cost cutting," and that great favorite "the bottom line" creep into inservice meetings and discussions. Our cries about understaffing fall on deaf ears. The budget, which was put on the back burner at the outset of the new era is, again, our master, one that must be honored and obeyed. Financial figures and statistics are hurtled at us with typhoon intensity. We dodge and weave, but the barrage is constant and unrelenting. We are slaves to terms that increase our misery and confusion, but definitely not our salaries.

"If we're going to get this, I'll have to check my budget for capital equipment. If I'm already over, I'll put it in for next year."

"According to corporate, we need to seek opportunities to reduce staffing by 2.5 full-time employees by the end of the fiscal year." It still sounds like layoffs to me.

Then the nurse manager disappears. In an effort to insure position and stature, the manager joins committees, lots of them. And goes to meetings. Lots of those, too. There are meetings to form new committees and committees that establish the where and when of the next meeting. Days go by and the manager is never seen. At the store, you search for her face on milk cartons. You wait for her story to appear on "Unsolved Mysteries."

When a disappearance act is so pronounced, it can also be regarded as a means of escape. Perhaps, the manager took on too much and doesn't know how to handle the problems plaguing the department. In committees, the nurse manager may be a star. Administration may see her as super, someone who definitely bears watching for advancement. In the meantime, her department is a disaster, the period of heroism has long since given way to one of dissatisfaction and disillusionment. Backstabbing is number one on the hit parade and morale has completely dropped of the chart. What happened?

Forgetting Our Roots

What happened was that the nurse manager forgot her roots. Courted and successfully wooed by the higher-ups, the manager conveniently forgot her past. What is more important is she forgot what it was like **to be a nurse.** At first, she was willing to remember. She might have even seen herself as a savior of sorts, someone who was well versed in the problems of her profession. She was going to right those wrongs, make the workplace a smooth running department. Issues would be confronted and resolved. She would wrestle with the devil and win.

However, in face-to-face combat with administration, she was made to see the error of her ways. Her superiors worked on her steadily to win her to their way of thinking. They worked their way around her with the idea that since she's a nurse, she'll be easy to manipulate. Their strategy is flawless, tried and well proven. Look around.

There is, on occasion, an exception: the maverick. This nurse manager is the answer to our prayers. This is the person who doesn't care about administration's philosophy. This is the manager who believes in the lessons and experiences of her past. She wants to run her department and be left alone. In turnabout, she uses the administration to meet her department's needs and achieve her goals. She doesn't own a silk suit and has no use for lab coats. She assesses the committees and the meetings and attends those that will allow her to do her job. At times, she will ignore administration and do things her way (watch out, big boys!). The staff in the department loves her. She is truly their advocate. She fights for them and takes on the problems as they come. There is little friction because matters that create dissension are disposed of efficiently. The doctors love her because she gets things done and is straightforward. She makes no excuses and she accepts none. As expected, she doesn't last. Once administration realizes there is a maverick in their midst, the plotting begins for the inevitable ouster. The maverick is replaced by a robot, a Stepford nurse manager.

"Do What I Say, Or Else!"/ We Don't Know How to Talk to Each Other

It is one of life's bitter ironies that nurses, who are taught from day one to speak with kindness and understanding to patients and with deference and respect to doctors, don't know how to speak to each other. This is especially evident in interactions between senior staff nurses/nurse managers and staff nurses. Besides forgetting their roots, nurses in authority often revel in their power and use it as a weapon rather than a tool.

"I'm the manager and I can do whatever I want."

"I'm the senior staff nurse and you'll do as I tell you."

"I never give breaks or lunches."

Unfortunately, such abuse of power often hearkens back to the time when those in authority were under similar thumbs. They have learned through the example of their predecessors. Worse yet, they are carrying on a tradition out of revenge. The thinking goes that, if I was treated this way, the day I have some clout I'm going to do the same thing. So, crazed with power, they stomp on everything and everyone in sight.

Nurse managers often take another tact when trying to elicit cooperation from the staff. More like "I am the mom and you are the kids," it is equally ineffective. This ploy also involves the guilt trip and tugging on those dedication strings.

At a time when it was impossible to shore up the evening shift in one hospital, the day shift was told they would be rotating through this shift ("Do what I say, or else!"). Because of the nature of the plan, hours would also be cut back. So the staff was experiencing not only the inconvenience of a surprise shift change, but also a reduction in work and pay. Furious at this arbitrary assignment, the nurses called a meeting with the manager, for the assignment created havoc with personal lives that relied on the consistency of definite working hours.

In the wake of this confrontation and upheaval, the nurse manager weakly explained her reasoning. She ended her comments with the assertion that she thought everyone would work together and pitch in at this difficult time. "Where is your sense of dedication? There was a time when everyone would help out." The staff pointed out that dedication didn't pay the mortgage or the groceries, and they were more interested in the tangible financial rewards of their profession.

Inevitably, there are times when managers accept absurd policies without question and try to inflict them on their departments. At one hospital where I worked, the administration decided to staff the OR on Saturdays, rather than have a call team available. This would save the hospital money, they reasoned. The idea was that two of us assigned to Saturdays would do the cases scheduled and remain in the hospital until the end of the shift. Instead of being available on a beeper for the rest of the shift, we were to use our time doing busy work.

"You can come in here," the nurse manager took us into the instrument room.

"You can dust the shelves and clean the cabinets," she continued.

I was incredulous.

"I have someone who comes to my home and does this," I responded. "If you need this kind of help, I'll be happy to send her down."

The manager just looked at me, stupefied. My point was beyond her comprehension, but I felt better. The mandatory Saturday shifts were short-lived once the higher-ups realized this new idea was not cost effective (in fact, it was more costly than the original on-call method).

The Iron Hand of Control

For some nurse managers, control is everything. Already closet control freaks, in their new position of authority, control not only comes out of the closet, but it also runs rampant in the halls. It's not enough to dominate the department, but their jurisdiction must extend to its every aspect. I know of one nurse manager so adamant that the radio filtering tunes throughout the building remain on the station she chose, that she fixed the receiver to prevent any channel adjustment.

The need to control evokes a great deal of game playing. Managers keep tabs on time spent on breaks and at lunch and use this as leverage to gain "cooperation" from staff. Managers displeased with staff members may deny vacation requests or harass employees about sick time. They threaten rather than cajole and are heavy-handed at any opportunity. Such nurse managers reward the meek and the martyrs. They squelch independent thought and suggestions and brand as troublemakers anyone who might disagree with them or with hospital/corporate policy.

Failure to relinquish any control produces workaholics. Administration smiles on these "dedicated" individuals, happy to have them on their team, in their corner. For these are the "company" people who are doggedly devoted to the institution and feel it cannot err. They believe the pabulum they are fed and are shocked when their staff does not. One health care corporation sent out a memo advising employees of forthcoming labor and non-labor "cost reduction opportunities." Employees were neither fooled nor charmed by this term. Morale decreased considerably as people discussed the possibility of layoffs. The manager regarded all this with a jaundiced eye and warned the employees not to spread rumors, for this alone could result in termination. The staff capitulated, muttering their discontent when the manager was out of sight.

Denial is another means of maintaining control. Should a facility be closing down, it is not unusual for management to deny this until the last minute. The rationale is that it averts panic. It also prevents employees from looking for other jobs. Recently, a rumor circulated in a facility that was constantly crying "Wolf!" about money that managers had been given a bonus. This followed a period of layoffs and cutbacks. When confronted with this rumor, a nurse manager denied it emphatically. However, the rumor persisted. Finally, another nurse manager met with her staff and verified that the rumor was true. Eventually, a memo was released by those sainted souls in plush, carpeted offices, acknowledging that bonuses had been distributed. Of course, the explanation was given in that special language of administrators: doubletalk.

Keep 'Em Down, Keep 'Em Humble

There are nurse managers who think the world of their nurses and let them know they're appreciated. Then there are those who think they do this, but actually do the opposite. In a continuing effort to control nurses, it is not extraordinary for managers to take a negative approach. That is, rather than tell employees how well they perform, they make it a point to tell the nurses what a lousy job they're doing. Sometimes this is a prelude to a compliment, but the ensuing compliment is lost when self-worth is already trashed. When confronted with the negative charge, the employees may want specifics and are further frustrated when they not given. One group of nurses, when told they didn't work together as a team, wanted examples. The senior staff nurse was unable to comply. The nurses' response was, "How can we correct a problem if we don't know the specifics? We think we do work as a team." Vague murmurings and vacant looks from the senior staff nurse were the only reply. The nurses were left angry and confused. Morale plummeted.

Nebulous accusations can be taken to an individual level as well. One nurse was taken aside by both the nurse manager and the senior staff nurse, who informed the unsuspecting person that several complaints had been brought to their attention by other members of the staff. Again, when specific incidents were requested, there were none that could be recalled. The nurse wanted to meet with her accusers. This opportunity was denied. The nurse was left to wonder not only about her own performance, but also whether to trust those with whom she worked. After years together, she wondered, why couldn't her co-workers speak directly to her about any problems they were noticing? These hide-and-seek tactics serve to keep the staff off guard and off balance. It keeps them looking over their shoulders and wondering what's next.

Trying to regulate a department in such a devious manner is extremely self-defeating. The control that is garnered is offset by a whopping and constant morale problem. Also employees are astute and wise to such tactics. Yet, unhappily, duplicity will still be mildly effective. Although nurses might be savvy to what's going on and tend to disregard it, a negative or accusatory comment will unwittingly strike dischord, creating the desired effect of keeping the staff off balance and under control.

Divide and Conquer: Dazed and Confused

For some nurse managers, nothing is more threatening than a department where everyone gets along. Therefore, another managerial ruse is to pit one employee against another, for a divided department has neither strength nor clout. This can be achieved by sending out mixed messages to different members of the staff. It also relies on poor communication and the fact that most women are nonconfrontational. This encourages backbiting and unrest. The more disruption, the better. You keep them down when you keep them guessing. It may not make for an efficient department, but it does create a controlled department or unit. The right hand not only doesn't know what the left hand is doing, but it doesn't care.

One means of dividing and conquering in particular departments is to have individuals who specialize in one job or procedure to the exclusion of all others. This method spawns little domains. While some nurses are willing to share their knowledge, there are others who aren't. They guard their areas of expertise with a vigilance worthy of the CIA, often to the extent that an intruder will be sabotaged. This might be achieved in the OR by hiding needed instruments, doctors' preference cards, or being unavailable as a resource person. The unwitting victim (who may have been reluctant to invade this sacred territory in the first place) is left to founder in the angry sea of orthopedics, neurosurgery or whatever and deal with the unchecked wrath of a doctor who stirs up the already tumultuous waters by saying, "These problems never occur when I work with ———." This sentiment will doubtless be taken to the department manager who will smile agreeably and see to it that ——— is back at his/her post immediately. Nurse V ("V" is for victim), who may have wanted to try something new, now retreats to a corner to patch her broken wings. Such is life in the land of the conquered.

Alone at the Top

The nurse administrator is one of the more interesting hospital phenomena. This is an individual stuck in a nether world, not really a nurse (in the true sense of the word) and not quite an administrator. It is perceived that the farther up the hierarchical ladder the nurse goes, the farther from the patient he or she is. This is true physically. Unhappily, this person is still stuck in the confines of being a nurse whose voice is conveniently ignored when she pleads for a larger budget for appropriate levels of staffing. Even at this exalted level, the nurse is controlled and still has no autonomy.

Nursing Organizations: What Are They Doing for Us?

The American Nurses Association, the National League of Nursing, state nurses' associations and those organizations specific to nursing specialties such as AORN (Association of Operating Room Nurses) offer a more positive side to the politics of nursing. While these organizations have their own political in-house squabbles and games and, while some of their undertakings may appear to be self-serving, these associations present a cohesive front of professionalism. They provide their membership with "the big picture" of nursing as a nationally recognized entity. Indeed, theirs is the unenviable task of pulling together the many disparate factions of nursing and motivating them to look beyond their own self-interests for the good of the profession as a whole.

The National League of Nursing serves as a nationwide educational entity, offering libraries of videos and books to individuals and institutions for self-improvement and continuing education. The League strives to keep nurses apprised of current practices and looks for changes that might alter the course of the profession in the future.

Meeting in June 1993, NLN's membership directed the organization to push for graduate degrees for nurses aspiring to advanced nursing practice. The League was also urged to "solicit federal funds for graduate education and to promote program models for both advanced practice nurses who don't hold graduate degrees and for degree-holding nurses who aren't now nurse practitioners" (*American Journal of Nursing*, November 1993).

The American Nurses Association is at the forefront in nationalizing issues that are or should be of concern to all nurses, irrespective of specialty. Recognizing that nursing has become increasingly more political, ANA works toward unifying the legions of nurses, working or retired, throughout the United States. The ANA works through the state nursing associations and very often levels its political clout through these SNAs. The ANA's efforts can be seen in strong educational programs and the steadfast lobbying of state and Congressional legislators to pass bills that will help nurses either personally, as wage earners, or professionally. "Among ANA's current issues are those which:

- ➢ Secure direct Medicare and Medicaid payment for nursing services.
- ➢ Recognize nursing as a revenue-generating service and reimburse nurses accordingly.

Most recently, ANA was instrumental in passage of the Rural Nursing Incentive Act, which provides direct Medicare payment to rural nurses for their services, and gives vital support to passage of community nursing and ambulatory care demonstration legislation. Other ANA-supported laws recognize nurses' rights to engage in collective bargaining" (taken from the ANA pamphlet *Nursing & the American Nurses Association).*

The ANA spent the better part of 1993 preparing nurses for health care reform. Looking to the future, the organization advocated that today's nurses and future nurses be directed to primary care. It emphasized that "education must focus on primary care and the management of acute minor illness and complex chronic diseases" (*American Journal of Nursing*, August 1993). In addition, "the House of Delegates took a strong stance on nurses' right to be involved in restructuring services and on the urgency of developing staffing methodologies reflecting 'professional nursing standards'."

The major vehicle of communication for the ANA is the *American Journal of Nursing (AJN)*, a slick publication that offers a bounty of information. State nursing and specialty associations also provide publications designed to keep their members informed of critical and current nursing issues. Never has this been more crucial than in this era of health care reform. This topic has been so fraught with controversy that the very mention of it has caused people's eyes to roll around uncontrollably, much the way Wile E. Coyote's do after an encounter with the Roadrunner and a load of dynamite.

The ANA (together with other nursing organizations) has formulated *Nursing's Agenda for Health Care Reform*. This is nursing's contribution to create "a health care system that assures access, quality, and services at affordable costs." The *Agenda*, (see Appendix A) calls for the following:

- ➢ a basic "core" of health care services to be available to everyone
- ➢ a restructured health care system that will focus on the consumers and their health, with services to be delivered in familiar, convenient sites, such as schools, workplaces, and homes
- ➢ a shift from the predominant focus on illness and cure to an orientation toward wellness and care

This *Agenda* was carefully thought out and represents an ambitious collective undertaking to bring to the attention of our legislators that nurses are here, and we're an integral part of health care so **pay attention to us and listen to what we have to say!!**

Like any other organization, the ANA is not without its flaws and its critics. It is, after all, a political organization and subject to the same idiosyncrasies that affect all political animals. Many nurses share the perspective that the ANA has caved in to the idea that unlicensed assistive personnel are here to stay. Accordingly, the association is trying to minimize the trauma by aligning itself with hospital administrators and offering the philosophy of making the best of a very poor situation. The result is the establishment of standards of practice for unlicensed assistive personnel; and the nurses delegated to supervise them. Harold Stearley, in his article, "Restructuring and the ANA: Whose Side are They on?" asserts that the ANA is attempting to mothball staff nurses in an effort to back up nursing administrators who "are using UAP to replace RNs in order to cut costs and protect their own inflated salaries." (*Revolution*, Fall 1994). Again, a lack of unity is all too evident. It's nurse against nurse as we compromise ourselves *again*.

Nurses have been so bogged down fighting among each other that those in the rank-and-file are being compromised. The circumstances are muddied by a lot of double talk, but the results are the same: layoffs, layoffs, layoffs. Health care reform has its own aberrant version of "trickle down economics:" all patients have primary care physicians who don't want to share their portion of the financial pie with specialists. So they treat their patients themselves until they absolutely **have** to refer to a surgeon, podiatrist, orthopedist, etc. Consequently, there are, for example, fewer surgeries. For nurses this translates into fewer patients on the wards, fewer operations (inpatient and outpatient), fewer nurses needed in the

OR, in ambulatory surgery, in post-anesthesia care units, in pre-op admission areas. Hours are cut. Positions are eliminated.

In California, which seems to be the prototype state for managed care, the woes of financial stress and/or ruin recently espoused by physicians are being taken to heart by nurses. As Professor Harold Hill warned the townspeople about their children in *The Music Man,* "Have you noticed that certain words are creeping into their vocabulary...?" In managed care, the "certain words" are "restructuring" and "redesigning" jobs and job opportunities. Nurses realize that health care reform is going to have a dramatic effect on our roles as patient advocates as well as wage-earners.

Suddenly, doctors and nurses find themselves on the same side of a financial battlefield that is affecting personal incomes as well as compromising patient care. Such an affiliation is somewhat unique considering the history of the doctor/nurse relationship.

CHAPTER FIVE

Doctors And Nurses: What's Going On Here Anyway?

Is History Repeating Itself?

It's a familiar scene: the older doctor, noble, and honorable, wearing a finely starched white lab coat over a Brooks Brothers suit, shirt and tie ensemble. This man of unquestionable character verily reeks of integrity. Picture, if you will, someone of the George C. Scott or Sean Connery genre. He (Yes, it's a *he;* we're dealing with stereotypes here!) personifies trust and caring. He is the venerable general practitioner or the gifted surgeon. There is no ego evident which is another degree of fantasy!

Enter the nurse. She is young, shapely, and dedicated. She wears her spotless white uniform with pride and conviction. When Dr. Marvelous approaches, she readily gives up her seat at the nurses' station and eagerly awaits the orders that will send her scurrying to the bedside of her patients. The verbal exchange is predictable:

"Good morning, honey," says Dr. M. "How are you today?"

"Just fine, Dr. Marvelous."

"Do you have the charts on my patients?" The doctor, places a protective arm around the nurse.

"Yes, doctor, they're right here," the nurse answers promptly.

A conversation most likely follows, wherein the nurse gives a report based upon information she received at the beginning of her shift, as well as what she has observed since coming to work. Dr. M. nods knowingly. The impression is that he is hearing, but is not listening. Finally, he gets up and makes rounds on his patients. As he leaves, he pats the nurse on the back and says, "You girls sure do a fine job." The nurse beams appreciatively, like an eager-to-please puppy, grateful for the acknowledgment. The scene fades, capturing the nurse's happy glow of recognition.

Until the last ten or fifteen years, such an encounter was not uncommon. Nightingale nurses, as we have seen, were taught in a stifling atmosphere of obedience and conformity. Their successors were taught in training to relinquish their chairs whenever a doctor arrived. Self-effacement was their hallmark and can still be seen in some nurses today. Nurses were referred to as "honey" or "dear" or "sweetie" as well as by their first names (if the noble physician could remember the nurse's first name). Nurses expected a condescending attitude from physicians, and assumed that their efforts, charting notes, and suggestions would be ignored if the physician was in a *good* mood.

If an order was not carried out or recorded, or if an order was questioned because of illegible writing (imagine that!) or if the doctor was in a foul mood, terms of familiarity were quickly replaced by terms of abuse. When problems arose with the care of the patient, it was (and, unfortunately, still is) not unusual for the doctor to point an accusing finger at the nurse.

If the patient's lab work wasn't done on time, it must have been the nurse's fault. Never mind that a power failure rendered the lab useless for four hours or that a bomb threat was called in to the hospital and the building had to be evacuated.

If the physician couldn't draw blood from the patient on the first attempt, it must have been the nurse's fault. After all, (s)he provided the dull needles, or the gloves that were too large, or the inadequate tourniquet that made the task impossible. That the patient was a longtime drug abuser or on ongoing chemotherapy, which made locating a vein extremely difficult, was not even a consideration.

If an operating room was running behind schedule, obviously it was because the nursing team moved like slugs. It couldn't be because the surgeon for the first case was late (no!) or the case was scheduled for one hour when three hours would have been more appropriate.

The nurse experienced and absorbed derision and, at times, personal attacks. There was never an attempt at self-defense; the nurse just "took it" even though a part of her died inside. Should the physician make a mistake, the chances of an apology were slim and none.

Father/Daughter—Husband/Wife

The relationship between doctors and nurses, hierarchical in nature, was similar to that of father and daughter. The wise physician kept a protective wing around the naïve and subservient handmaiden who obeyed his orders and followed his advice. These roles were shaped by gender and training. After all, nursing was considered women's work. Recommendations coming from a nurse required psychological acrobatics so that the physician would see a suggestion as his innovation. So fragile was the ego of the doctor, that any advice or proposal from an inferior nurse was regarded as insulting or belittling. That was then; this is now.

The father/daughter relationship has been altered considerably, definitely to the advantage of nurses. No longer willing to accept the doctor as infallible, nurses are learning to rely on our own experience, expertise, and education to question calls made by doctors. Nurses do not hesitate to make recommendations. Best of all, we nurses are learning to stand up for ourselves and to defend ourselves against humiliating verbal beatings. Sticking with the stereotype for one more sentence, it's safe to say that the father/daughter relationship is gradually evolving to more of a husband/wife relationship. This is due, in part, to burgeoning respect physicians feel toward nurses, who are also taking a stand against physician tyranny whenever possible. Doctors now work *with* nurses instead of barking orders. Now there is team effort. Recommendations are considered and doctors discuss with nurses what will benefit their patients. Much to their credit (although it was a long time coming), doctors are listening to what nurses are saying and relying on their information.

It is not coincidental that this new equality has come along when the demographics in medicine and nursing are changing. Today, it can no longer be assumed that the doctor will be a man and the nurse, a woman. As of 1993, 42% of freshman medical students were women. In 1994, 38.1% of students graduating from medical school were women. Among practicing physicians, women comprise 19.4%, not an overwhelming statistic, but one that is increasing.

In medicine, women physicians had to fight for their rights. They became assertive and aggressive, as necessary, to achieve their goals and attain the status they justly deserved. These women physicians know the difficulties of being a woman in a world populated and, at times, overrun by men, and they are ever respectful of the hardworking nurse. Women physicians know how helpful nurses can be to the learning physician and, undoubtedly, on their road to private practice, they have developed good working relations with nurses.

While only 6.2% of practicing nurses are male, more men are finding nursing an appealing profession. Although salaries are not high, nursing offers stability and mobility, and extra shifts can augment emergency financial needs.

In the 1970s, following the Vietnam war, men who were trained as medics often turned to nursing. Since that time, nursing programs have seen the number of male entry-level students increase to 9.5%, according to a June 1992 article in the *American Journal of Nursing*. The article further discloses that 5.2% of all RNs returning for college degrees are men.

Male nurses add another dimension to medicine; they fit easily into the "good ol' boy" network. As in the business world, it is not unusual for male nurses (especially senior staff nurses or nurse managers) and male physicians to resolve their differences and reach understandings on the golf course or on the ski slopes. At times, this camaraderie extends to sales representatives from medical supply companies. Without a doubt, the magic of male bonding is making the world a safer place for all of us!

My Name Is…

While the disparity between doctors and nurses is closing, there are still significant gaps that prevent the breach from being resolved quickly. Nowhere is this more evident than in the manner in which the groups address each other. Inevitably, nurses are Susies, Marys, Joes, and Garys. Nurses claim that it is easier for patients to know them by first names only. We are a blur of single names on the telephone and in person:

"Four South, Sue speaking."

"Surgery. This is Joan."

"My name is Jerry. I'll be your nurse today."

We are paged throughout our departments by our first names only:

"Debbie, you have a call on line one."

"Marty, please call extension 7232."

On a daily basis, we float in and out of patients' rooms and lives, indistinguishable beings in a continuous round of treatments.

Physicians, on the other hand, impress immediately with a full name and title. They are not concerned with confusing the patient with a complicated last name. Rather, they want to be sure the patient knows it and knows it well, especially when the time comes to pay the bill!!

The double standard of the familiar versus the formal perpetuates the subservient image of nurses. Writer Suzanne Gordon notes that it delivers "a very heavy message about who is and who is not a professional, a grown-up, and in charge in the institution in which they work" (*Revolution*, Fall 1993). Ms. Gordon continues by emphasizing that when nurses refer to other nurses by first names when speaking with a patient, yet persist in using a physician's title and last name, they are saying "that doctors are the only memorable, important players on the health care stage, and nurses are only handmaidens and physicians' helpers." These status lessons are magnified "each time nurses do this on television, in specials, or in news reports on health care issues."

Conversely, Gordon states, doctors and nurses who refer to each other by first names in front of patients send two vital messages: "...that their doctor is not a god, and... that nurses and doctors are collaborators and colleagues, rather that subordinate and superior."

"You **@@##*!"/ "Yes, Doctor!"

"When I was a resident my attending, Dr. X, was a notorious jerk," a surgeon told me once. "One time he reached up on the Mayo stand to grab his own instruments and the scrub nurse tapped him on the hand to remind him not to do that. His response was to take the entire Mayo tray and throw it across the room." It was not to the storyteller's credit that he found the entire episode amusing and justifiable.

What the scrub nurse had done was neither unusual nor out of line. It is one of the unwritten rules of surgery that the doctor asks for what he needs and he keeps his hands off the

Mayo stand. In fact, many surgeons apologize for reaching for their own instruments or ask if they might do so.

Fending for oneself goes with the territory for operating room nurses. However, at times, matters do get out of hand. As recently as February 1995, the *American Journal of Nursing* reported the following:

> Shot with a surgical staple gun by a surgeon who said it was a joke, a New Orleans nurse was awarded $5,000 by a jury. She fared better than a New Mexico OR nurse who was jabbed in the back with a bone chisel; in that case, an appellate court reasoned that a finding of assault requires a threat that puts the victim on notice of danger. The court dismissed the charge because it saw no evidence that the nurse had expected the surgeon to assault her (p. 76).

Physicians take their frustrations and insecurities out on the staff, the building and the instruments. I heard of one doctor who threw a syringe across a room with such force that the attached needle was imbedded in the wall. Another surgeon, irritated by the dullness of a pair of his own scissors, sent them flying across the room, almost hitting a nurse. On another occasion, a doctor picked up a nurse and hurled *her* against the wall, breaking her glasses.

Stories abound about the tirades of surgeons, their screaming fits and insulting verbal assaults. Nurses have been called "dummies" or "stupid" or worse. We are frequently reminded of our insignificance and that the doctor guarantees our jobs by bringing his or her patients to our facility. A doctor once told me that I should thank him for giving me job security.

Unfortunately, the healing hand is also a punishing hand. Some physicians are caught up in a cycle of violence not unlike that found in abusive homes. Their behavior, however, is learned in medical school. A survey of 431 medical students reported in 1991 revealed that 46% of the surveyed students and 81% of the seniors had experienced abuse in medical school (*Nursing Management*, March 1991).

The medical student ultimately becomes a physician who continues the cycle of humiliation and degradation. Now, the individual on the receiving end, in many cases, is the nurse. The result is painful and engenders feelings of worthlessness, powerlessness and poor self-image. A 1989 survey of 459 nurse managers and 709 staff nurses showed that 97.1% of nurse managers and 96.7% of staff nurses experienced verbal abuse (*Nursing Management*, March 1991). More than 85% of the respondents felt that verbal abuse contributed to errors and staff turnovers.

Nurses have responded to such insults with passive acceptance and indirect expressions of anger (lashing out at the first poor innocent to come along, be it colleague, husband, child, family dog, or goldfish). Most frequently, the emotions realized are fear, anger, anxiety, and frustration. However, the days of passive tolerance are slipping away and, finally, nurses are beginning to stand up to physicians.

Today, verbal and nonverbal outbursts are usually handled carefully, tactfully, and directly. Going one-on-one with a doctor will sometimes only serve to make a bad situation worse. If a patient is in jeopardy (which may have triggered the initial outburst), the matter is best handled by silence. There will be time enough to resolve the matter at the end of the crisis. If a nurse isn't comfortable confronting the physician, he or she may ask the department supervisor to do so instead. If this isn't feasible, the nurse might want to send the doctor a letter, with copies going to the immediate manager and the chief of the medical staff. Some facilities have methods for "writing up" offenders so that they are reprimanded appropriately

Sexual harassment is also part of the doctor/nurse game. A physician asked a nurse to bend over so that he could look down her scrub shirt. "I'm horny," he offered by way of an explanation. "Go home to your wife then," she suggested. Another doctor, commenting on a nurse's obvious weight loss, reminded her that now she "had no tits." The nurse sent him a letter, with a copy going to her department manager; the doctor received "counseling" from the hospital's personnel department.

During a surgery performed by two surgical residents, a man and a woman, the woman was explaining how much she enjoyed cardiovascular surgery. She especially liked the feel of the cardiovascular needle holders in her hand. "Oh," replied her colleague. "Did it give you an orgasm?" The woman physician pointed out the inappropriateness of this comment and concluded that she would be justified in "writing him up" for being so offensive. The circulating nurse agreed and ultimately wrote up the surgeon who was counseled and told that further such behavior could jeopardize his career.

In all fairness, it must be acknowledged that nurses use their own forms of harassment as a means of getting even. When working with an especially abusive surgeon, one operating room nurse made it a point to stay well within his peripheral vision throughout the case. She knew this irritated him and she took great pride in working out a strategy that allowed her a method of revenge. Ideally, egos and personal grudges should be put aside when caring for the patient, but that's like wishing some people would leave their personalities in the parking lot.

Untoward events of abuse and harassment tend to dismiss the final effect on the person at the bottom of the totem pole—the patient. However, patients are finding that they can fend for themselves especially since they hold the purse strings. They are the ones who enable the physician to afford his mortgage and car payment. That can be very effective leverage in dealing with the medical deities. One patient who heard her physician railing while she was awaiting surgery called him over and told him that she would cancel the procedure if he didn't quit yelling and calm down.

Patients may inadvertently be at the bottom of the medical stack, but like the acrobat who supports a ladder of three acrobats on his shoulders, the patient is crucial to the system.

Changing the Rules of the MD/RN Game

Just when doctors were getting comfortable in the doctor/nurse game, one of the sides changed the rules. Surprise! Nurses don't want to play any more. At least not according to the original and antiquated rules, carved in stone and presented to medicine by "Doctor Moses." As Howard Cosell said years ago on Monday Night Football, "Parity has come to the NFL." So, too, has parity emerged in medicine. The cause of this parity is education.

More and more, nurses are graduating from colleges and universities with bachelor degrees in nursing. Many go on to get masters' degrees and doctorates. Physicians with 8-10 years of education and training are now working with nurses who have 4-9 years of college education, rather than a nurse who has completed only three years of training in nursing school.

The deferential handmaidens of the past are being replaced by specialty trained, advanced practitioners. We perform our duties as independently as possible, and we are directly responsible to patients. We resent oldline nurses who want to remain bogged down in their prehistoric philosophies and handmaiden personae. They are barriers not only to themselves, but also to the rest of us who are trying to bring nursing into the 21st century. Younger nurses, who are better educated and willing to take chances, are saying, "This doctor/nurse game is ridiculous. We're outta here!" They start their own businesses, go back to school to major in something other than nursing; or (Oh, my!) become lawyers!

Nurses are demanding the autonomy and respect that befits highly educated individuals and *finally,* physicians are listening. Doctors are acknowledging that nurses deserve recognition and that they had better jump on the bandwagon or they will be run over by it! As Bob Dylan said in *The Times They Are A'Changin'*: ". . .he who gets hurt, will be he who has stalled. . ."

Yet, the doctor/nurse battle isn't the only one in town. We nurses must also look over our shoulders so that we can cover our backsides as we prepare to do battle with that ever-present adversary: hospital administration.

CHAPTER SIX

Hospitals And Nurses: The Battle Inside Raging

Tripping Over the Bottom Line

Hospitals are businesses. Their ultimate goal is to make money. If they don't make money, they don't stay in business. How else can you explain Sacred Heart General Hospital in Eugene, Oregon spending $65,000 to install an espresso bar while nurses and other employees are being laid off? "It's good business sense," explained a hospital spokesperson.

Originally small community havens for the sick and dying, hospitals are now big business. Metropolitan areas that once boasted of many independent facilities now find themselves in the middle of turf wars as the more powerful (read: wealthier) facilities grab smaller independents and make them part of the conglomerate. Inevitably, a "parent" company oversees activities for an entire region and monitors faltering hospitals seeking the right opportunity to bail them out and make them part of the corporate family.

Hospitals are medical bureaucracies whose goals are to conduct business as efficiently as possible. We nurses do not do well in a bureaucratic setting that tends to clash with our professional values. We are compelled to follow the edicts and directives of those higher up the ladder—physicians and administrators—who expect unflagging loyalty and devotion (do *not* question authority). As hospitals struggle under various financial obligations, nurses are worked to death, burnt out, and looking for a better deal. The irony here is that even with layoffs and "restructuring," there is still a nursing shortage and hospitals are scrambling to replace those who were "restructured" out onto the street. Agencies still receive desperate calls for "quick fix" staffing for departments where workloads remain heavy. Staffing properly remains a troublesome quandary that leaves departments foundering, patients poorly attended, and nurses exhausted.

The competition for hospitals is fierce; the pace is frenetic. To remain competitive, hospitals seek the latest in equipment and technology. They also look for every opportunity to reduce costs and increase profits. Hospital stays have been decreasing ever since Medicare came out with DRGs (Diagnosis Related Groups) ten years ago. The focus is now on outpatient care, where procedures are performed and the patient can go home the same day. The focus is also on reduced staff. "Downsizing" is the euphemistic term tossed about by business and the media, but if you're a nurse it translates into unemployment.

Where Have All the Nurses Gone?

In the spring of 1989, a young woman hospitalized with a pneumothorax (collapsed lung) hit the nurse call button to get assistance in repositioning herself in bed. A small indwelling chest tube used to alleviate her condition made moving quite painful. The patient waited and waited and waited. Finally, a scratchy voice screeched over the bedside intercom, the voice mail of the nursing station.

"Yes? What do you need?"

"I need help turning," came the reply.

"Well, there's no one around right now. It'll probably be a while."

"Forget it," answered the patient in exasperation. "I'll manage on my own."

Remote control nursing was, and still seems to be the rule, rather than the exception. Nurses are tuning in to reality, turning on to other careers and dropping out of their profession. In addition, nursing schools are realizing a 20% drop in enrollments. What happened? Apparently, several things occurred at roughly the same time.

There was always an attrition due to job burnout. However, in the late 1980s, job burnout was coupled with a change in job demographics as nurses opted to work in ambulatory centers, clinics, and home health care. These jobs offered a fairly normal schedule with no weekends or shift changes.

Nurses became more fed up as our responsibilities increased and our autonomy and salaries didn't. We started looking around for a better way to make a living and a better way of life.

In conjunction with this change in attitude, the image of nursing was catching up with the realities of the profession. High school students looked at the long hours, demanding tasks, and mediocre pay then said "Forget it! I'm going to be a senator!" Girls benefitted from the women's movement and saw that any numbers of avenues were available to them. Why should they go in for something with little glory and unending hassles? Why should a woman choose to be on the losing end of the doctor/nurse game when one can go to medical school and come out a winner?

Finally, hospitals and their administrations can be held responsible for the drastic number of turnovers and the shortage of nurses. By failing to understand and work with nurses in matters of concern, hospitals overwhelmingly contribute to this plight. In their article "The Nurse Shortage: Myth or Reality?," nurses Linda Aiken and Connie Mullinix state: "The fact is that nursing shortages are a consequence of complacent management and the reluctance of administrators to reexamine traditional practices" (*New England Journal of Medicine*, September 3, 1987).

We are experiencing a medical "Catch 22." Nurses leave nursing, very often because of attitudinal constipation on the part of hospitals. The hospital hierarchies weep, moan, and gnash their administrative teeth over being shortstaffed along with the difficulties of working within a claustrophobic budget. Yet, it is the hospital administrators, plagued by self-inflicted myopic vision, who have created the insane shortstaffing situation.

Are We Really Shortstaffed or Is It My Imagination?

Nursing surveys consistently reveal that understaffing is a top concern among nurses throughout the country.

Being shortstaffed is nothing new to nurses. It has long been a way of life. It seems that since time immemorial, there has been a nursing shortage, with the situation reaching critical proportions in the late 1980s. Today, it appears that shortstaffing is contrived by hospitals that are "restructuring" in an attempt to stem rising costs. The nurses are available, we just aren't being hired. In fact, many of us are being laid off.

There is little recourse available to nurses as we continue to struggle with long hours, inadequate help, and the current plague: unlicensed assistive personnel—individuals with meager education and little or no experience who must be monitored by an RN. Overworked and overwhelmed, nurses file complaints with management about such unacceptable work situations. While a nurse will not necessarily be fired for refusing an assignment or filing a complaint, there might be other repercussions. Vacations may be denied, or the individual may be assigned heavy loads on holidays and weekends. Refusal to perform assigned tasks (regardless of safety concerns) is seen as a lack of cooperation and will be an issue for discussion during that wonderful annual event: the performance evaluation. Here, it will be in writing for all the world to see: "Nurse Freethinker is uncooperative and difficult. Individual does not help when department is shortstaffed."

Some of us, who have the shelter of a bargaining unit (approximately 7% out of 2.2 million nurses) can design contracts to protect ourselves in shortstaffing arenas. Those of us who are not covered by such an umbrella must look to other resources to alter this unfortunate trend. It is imperative that we document our concerns, work together with our colleagues, professional organizations, and state nursing boards. Unless we speak out, no one will be aware of these ongoing problems and the repercussions that are having devastating effects on the nurses and our patients.

The National Nurse Survey (*Revolution*, Summer 1993) reported the following problems caused by understaffing:

Health care administrators are misusing nurses and their skills.

Despite understaffing and shortages of licensed nurses, administrators are increasing non-nurse duty assignments. On the average, one-fourth of a nurse's time on the job is spent removing trash, picking up meal trays, changing linens, and doing clerical work. This usually occurs because ancillary help has been reassigned or laid off to save money.

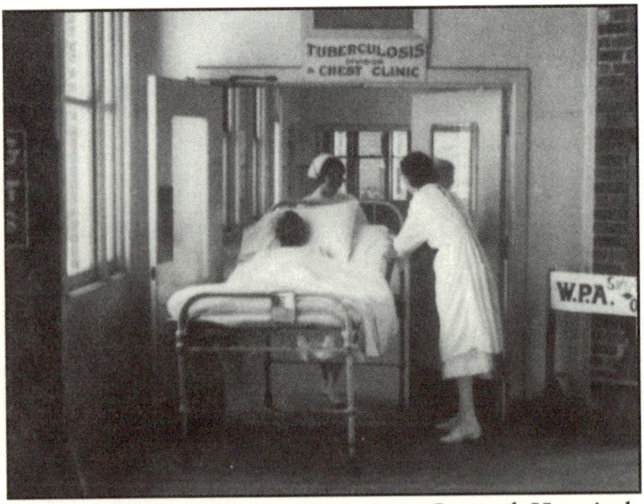

Turburculosis ward, San Francisco General Hospital, c. 1936. Transporting patients is one of several areas where, even today, nurses are used rather than ancillary personnel. (Courtesy UCSF archives.)

Quality of patient care is compromised.

Nurses don't have enough time to spend with their patients, thus patient-care tasks are neglected and serious accidents can occur. Official injury and accident statistics do not accurately reflect growing problems because nurses are able to report only half of the incidents created by shortstaffing. Error rates on shortstaffed units are double those on adequately staffed units. In one incident a patient accidentally drank formalin after a critical procedure had been performed and died because there was no one nearby to prevent this. Also, let's not forget the the recent "mistakes" (incorrect leg amputated, wrong patient removed from a respirator) at University Community Hospital in Tampa, Florida. The Health Care Financing Administration cited "staffing problems—including allowing unsupervised staff with minimal training to treat critically ill patients, and overloading nursing supervisors with other jobs that left them unable to supervise—as factors that contributed to the hospital's recent egregious mistakes" (*The American Nurse,* June 1995, p. 18).

Shortstaffing causes abnormally high rates of stress and stress-related illnesses among nurses.

The frustration and anxiety of dealing with understaffing continuously are realized in hypertension, depression, and ulcers, as well as other diseases. All of this eventually leads to burnout. Two out of three nurses indicate that they are ready to either leave their current posts or abandon the profession entirely.

Hospital administrators are using shortsighted personnel policies.

To compensate for the skeletal staffing, hospitals have developed innovative and creative staffing procedures. The in-house pool and "floating" are two such fascinating examples. Administrators think it works; we know it doesn't.

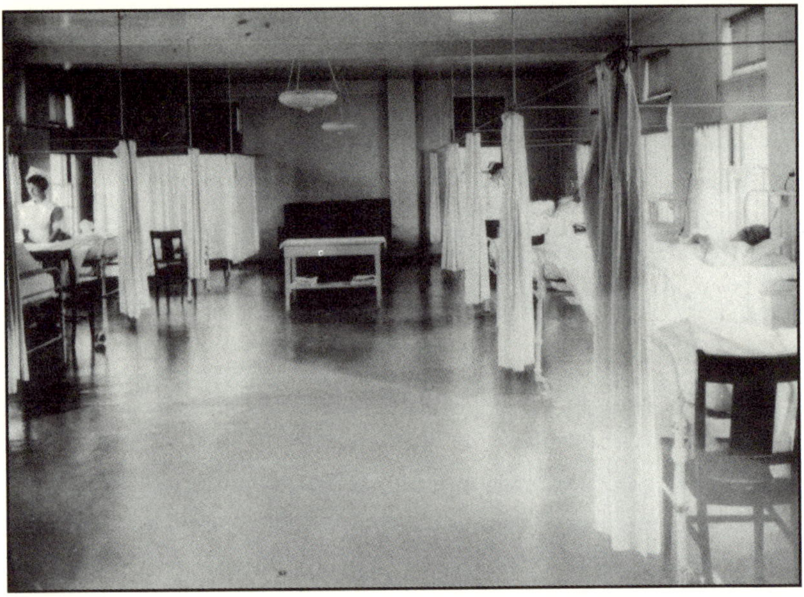

Men's ward, San Francisco General Hospital c. 1950. Shortstaffing compromises patient care. If this picture were taken today, the nurse would either be absent or replaced by an unlicensed individual. (Courtesy UCSF archives.)

The In-House Pool

In the last few years, hospitals have used the in-house pool as a means of providing an incentive for nurses to work additional hours or shifts. The procedure may vary with each institution, but the concept is basically the same. Nurses are offered more money (time-and-a-half plus a set dollar amount per hour) to work more. It is hoped that this incentive will encourage part-time employees and full-time employees to crank out some extra time, thereby eliminating the need to hire additional nurses (and pay benefits) or resort to the use of expensive nursing agency personnel. This is a dandy way to stretch the staff and speed up the burnout process.

To Float or Not to Float? That Is the Question

Another method of dealing with shortstaffed areas is to float nurses to different units. This has long been an area of controversy for nurses who find themselves in units where their expertise is minimal. A nurse from a medical floor who is sent to do a shift in a Coronary Care Unit may find the need for the unit's services herself once she gets a glimpse of the monitors and machines, which seemingly require a degree from MIT to operate and maintain.

Unless you and I have a specific agreement with our employer to the contrary, we are obliged to "float" as we are told. That is, we are happy swimmers in the **mandatory** float pool. As hospitals have become megacompanies with several facilities and campuses, floating has broadened to an inter-facility phenomenon. This is sort of a medical cross-pollination experience.

Imagine this scenario: you are happily employed at hospital A. It was your choice to work there. However, hospital A is having financial woes and the ever-invisible board of directors and administrators, together with a few token physicians (who probably do nothing but thoughtfully rub their chins during meetings) opt to put the hospital on the block. After much behind-the-scenes negotiating and amid flying rumors, an agreement is reached with those crafty diplomats from the local hospital industry. Hospital A is gobbled up with the enthusiasm of a Monopoly player purchasing Park Place or Boardwalk. Suddenly, Hospital A along with hospitals B, C and D is considered a happy family. Guess what? You're part of this cozy picture, too. Congratulations! You get to float all over town to these other hospitals. How is your anxiety level? Are you happy in your work?

It stands to reason that, if you had wanted to work at any of the other hospitals, you would have applied for a job there. However, for whatever reason, you didn't. It doesn't matter; you get to work there now. No big deal, the more optimistic part of you thinks. Change is good and at least you'll have your job. This is all very true. However, the same shortstaffing problems that you found difficult and ulcer-making in your home-away-from-home seem all the more glaring when you are in a strange place, particularly if you have no desire to be there in the first place. There are also other considerations.

An operating room nurse may find herself assigned to a procedure that was not performed in her home hospital or required to use equipment that may be completely different. An ambulatory surgery nurse may be assigned to a craniotomy or a thoracotomy. A floor nurse may be sent to intensive care, labor and delivery, or to the emergency room When a concern is voiced, the response might be "Well, you've done this before, haven't you?" This is true, but it was several years ago. "No problem. I'll send so and so in to help you." Never mind that the helper elf is deep in the heart of a ruptured aneurysm and hasn't seen the light of day (or the bathroom!) for hours. Any further concerns that are voiced will be perceived as complaining and unwillingness to help and will likely be brought up in (you guessed it!) the annual performance review.

Saying "No" and Paying the Price

So now what do you do? You drop back and punt, act like a martyr and go about your business. Or, you can take some action (you are such a troublemaker!).

If you just say "No," you can be fired unless a contract to the contrary exists between you (or your bargaining unit) and the hospital. Great, huh? Don't be discouraged. There are ways to make a difficult situation less so.

If the senior staff nurse is creating difficulties, go talk to the supervisor. Explain that you're here to help and you want to do a good job, but it would certainly be in the best interest of the department and the patient if you were assigned to do a procedure that you had performed in the past. It's essential that a resource be available and that there is a proper orientation to the unit. After all, we're supposed to be helping the patients, not risking their lives to save a buck.

Finally, nurses need to take an active role in the matter. In her article, "Floating," Marcia Lepler states: "Nurses must insist upon full participation in the development of floating policies and staffing formulas...They must continue to advocate for policies designed to minimize the necessity for floating and the liability associated with it" (*Revolution*, Spring 1993, p. 97).

When asked to float to a new, unfamiliar area, the nurse should assess the situation. If she is uncomfortable, she must alert the supervisor right away. Barbara Eileen Calfee, J.D., L.S.W. makes other recommendations: "negotiate a safe floating situation, submit a 'protest of assignment' form and make a private notation of the occurrence in a diary or journal" (*Revolution*, Spring 1993, p. 97).

Administration and Nursing: Oil and Water

Nurses have tried and continue to try to work with employers to resolve the shortstaffing issues. Sandy Houglin, manager for the center for labor work place advocacy at the American Nurses Association, states: "Nurses say it's (end of shortstaffing) just not going to happen, because the employer is either hard of hearing, or driven so much by the bottom line dollar that they don't care what the nurses think." Ms. Houglin continues by saying, "There is a perception out there that if it is coming from nurses, it can't be taken too seriously" (*Revolution*, Summer 1993, p. 12).

Overwork, understaffed areas and inappropriate floating can also lead to errors and poor patient care, which translates into lawsuits against the facility (remember the Florida hospital?). This realization is slowly sinking in, but the important thing is that the budget looks good and the bottom line smiles back at the honchos. Anyway, hospital corporations have legal firms on hefty retainers; so now the lawyers will be earning their money. Isn't it great how it all works out?!

CHAPTER SEVEN

Health Care And Nurses: Are We Losing Ground?

Here Comes Hillary! There Goes Hillary!

Our health care system is a mess and we are in dire need of reform. Millions of Americans are uninsured either because they are unemployed or because they are self-employed and can't afford hefty insurance payments that provide limited benefits. HMOs and managed care, with its capitation philosophy, dictate who we will see when we are sick. Emphasis on cost-cutting has left the very ill in the care of individuals who have very little training and limited, if any, experience. A blunt approach is often the most effective. Now that we know we're dealing with a health care disaster, we can continue trudging through the 1990s.

The subject of our faltering health care delivery system has been dissected, buried, and exhumed for further inspection. Thousands of participles have been dangled, infinitives split, i's dotted and t's crossed in an effort to bring the huddled masses up-to-date be they in Kansas City or Altoona. We know it's a disaster and we know the Clinton administration, via Hillary, put together an ambitious package. Should the package ever be resurrected and get through Congress, it will probably not even remotely resemble the original plan. There will be enough volleying ("We could do it this way." "Oh no, let's try it this way." "Well, what if we eliminate this and add that?" "I've got a better idea...") of Hillary's or anyone's proposal and suggested alternates to leave the nation's citizens reeling.

My initial response is to ignore pros, cons and any other information that might be meaningless fifteen seconds after it's uttered and wait for the final story to appear on the cover of *Time*. However, as a member of the health care profession, I need to be aware of the possibilities that are being entertained so that I have an idea of how I might be affected.

As expansive as health care reform is, there are several ideas being examined as possible avenues. Each will affect nurses in terms of their stature as professionals and their status as consumers (Will nurses still be able to bring home the bacon or will they be doing the unemployment shuffle?).

However, before we surge ahead on the reform bandwagon, it's important to realize what is happening in hospitals right now. The patient population has changed significantly during the past ten years. Inpatients are very sick. Some are chronically ill; others are terminally ill. Surgical procedures are performed on high risk patients—the elderly, those with chronic heart and/or lung disease, diabetes, etc. There are fewer patients, but they all require extensive, expensive care. Gone are the days when one was hospitalized for a hernia operation or a breast biopsy. Many procedures and much of the care that was once administered on an inpatient basis is now handled in the office of the primary care physician or in an ambulatory surgery center.

These new changes have also necessitated a shift in the focus of health care to age-related diseases from childhood illnesses. There is a stronger emphasis on wellness and the prevention of disease, as well as life extension. As baby boomers head for middle age, medicine is looking at mid-life crises, along with problems associated with stress and substance abuse. Since people are playing as hard as they work, there is also emphasis on fitness, leisure, recreation, and sports medicine for those weekend warriors.

During the last two to five years, California and Massachusetts have been in the throes of pioneering managed care and managed competition. As these terms are bandied about, the rest of the nation regards the pioneers without envy and wishes that this bi-coastal peek into the future would go away. It won't, so let's face the devil and see what this is all about.

Managed competition is the darling of Washington D.C. politicos and was the basic premise for the Clinton health plan. The idea is to establish networks (Regional Health Alliances), which would compete to sell all-encompassing health insurance packages that meet government criteria. It is "...a scheme that would essentially corporatize health care, and give the insurance industry almost total control of the nation's health care system," according to Suzanne Gordon in her article "Health care Reform—How 'The System' Works Against Nurses" (*Revolution,* Fall 1993).

Managed care pays a primary care physician a specific amount (capitation) whether or not the patient is treated. Cost containment is achieved by having only the primary care physician administer to all the patient's needs. Patients are referred to specialists only in dire emergencies. After all, why pay more money to a specialist when the general practitioner is already getting a set fee, irrespective of the treatment. Cost containment is the overriding factor, rather than quality of care.

The final option being tossed around is the idea of a single-payer system, much like that in Canada. In the Canadian system, there is public administration and accountability, and all providers are treated equally. Insurance companies are no longer a part of health care and, as they are run out of town, they take their mountains of paperwork and administrative costs with them. With this option, quality of patient care is the primary concern. The downside is that since the government administers the plan, Canadians must wrestle with the bureaucracy and the ever-present red tape.

All of these possibilities have created a rumor mill second only to that generated by the O.J. Simpson trial proceedings. Everyone knows something and, in some cases, what they don't know, they make up. Anxieties and stress levels are up, and so are the stocks of the companies that make Prozac and Valium!

This Reality Check Is Brought To You By The CNA

In June 1994 the California Nurses Association took the bull by the horns by publishing the "Top 10 Myths about Hospital Restructuring and Health Care Reform" (*California Nurse*, June 1994). Each myth was presented and rebutted individually. Some of the myths dealt with health care reform in general, while others addressed those concerns specific to nurses. Chief among these were:

Hospitals must cut costs because they are losing money.

Forbes magazine reported in January 1994 that health care has been the most profitable industry in the country over the past few years. For the first nine months of 1993, hospitals had their greatest operating margin since 1986, according to the American Hospital Association.

Declining hospital utilization demonstrates the financial crisis for hospitals.

Managed care plans guarantee revenue whether the service is used or not. Capitation provides a fixed fee, usually based on the patient's diagnosis or membership in a managed care plan, regardless of the actual length of stay or treatment provided. Kaiser, the nation's largest managed care Health Maintenance Organization, is also distinguished for the lowest hospitalization rates in the nation. Kaiser made $848 million in profits in 1993. Finally, when the census is low, hospitals also send home. . .employees, regardless of whether or not they are being reimbursed for those empty beds. This sharply cuts their labor costs, as well as reduces ancillary costs on supplies and food.

RNs and other hospital employees are the main reason for skyrocketing health care costs.

Employee wage and benefit costs as part of hospital budgets have actually fallen dramatically the past three decades. In 1962, labor costs accounted for 67% of hospital expenditures. By 1992, the percentage was below 54% for the same expenses.

By contrast, administrative costs, now a quarter of all hospital spending, have risen by 180% since 1968. Capital expenditures rose by 36% in the 1980s. Prescription drug costs have risen at three times the inflation rate and health insurance premiums increased to twice the inflation rate in the past decade.

Downsizing effectively reduces health care costs with no effects on patient care.

Downsizing can have deadly consequences. A national study of 281 hospitals issued in November 1993, found that hospitals that reduced their staffing by eight percent or more were 400 times more likely to experience an increase in patient illness and mortality rates.

Decreased use of RNs does not harm patient care.

Thirteen recent studies have documented that hospitals with a higher percentage of RNs have lower mortality rates (back to Florida!).

In 1989, *Hospitals* magazine asked 663 hospital chief executive officers to rank ten factors that most contribute to hospital quality. Nursing care was ranked at the top, even above physician care (isn't that a switch?!).

Despite mounting evidence to the contrary, hospitals continue to operate from a panicky perspective. Caught up in the morass of trendy financial chaos, hospitals cast about for the life preservers that will keep them afloat. This is a tricky situation since medicine and business are not soul mates in any sense of the term.

How to Succeed in Business...

Hospitals, as noted previously, fancy themselves to be corporations. They have their organization charts and flowcharts in place and they are ready to play with the big boys—almost. They still need some outside help. Recognizing that business is not their first area of expertise, hospitals have enlisted the help of experts. In many instances, they have called upon those megabuck honchos: consultants. Administrators glance around them and perceive their worlds to be in turmoil. They want to do something, but what? It's definitely time for the "restructuring police."

Let the Games Begin!

In her article, "PCAs & CTAs: Are They the Beginning of the End for Nursing?" (*Revolution,* Summer 1994), Bernice Buresh presents a very forthright picture of the role of consultants in "restructuring" as she quotes CNA's Chuck Idelson:

"Restructuring is being planned not by people who have experience in healthcare, but in business....They're conducting these changes as a way to increase the hospital's share of profits. We all know that health care costs are out of control. But the percentage of expenses spent on employee wages has declined in the last 20 years. The increases are attributable to administrative costs, insurance and pharmaceutical industry profits, physician self referral, waste and duplication of technology."

Ms. Buresh speaks to the claims of many consulting companies that have positioned themselves to profit from the current health care fiasco. American Practices Management, Inc. is a company in New York that "claims to have helped some 80 hospitals trim a total of $1 billion in expenses." This company and many other consulting wizards offer a whole new vocabulary "that accentuates the image of efficiency and attention to patients, and eliminates any hint of a negative outcome or profit incentive." Now we have these nifty little expressions sneaking into our every day conversation like "Operation Excellence" and "patient-focused care." However, these euphemisms do not aptly describe the potential havoc that lays in store for both nurses and patients.

This Is the Nurse Call Button—Good Luck!

In the brave new world of health care change, the primary customer of the hospital is no longer the patient. Rather, it is the managed care companies that receive the reverential nod from the hospital big shots. "...primary care providers are gatekeepers who do the bidding of their corporate employers," noted Suzanne Gordon in her article "R.N.s Beware! Health care 'Reform' May Give your Job to a Tech!" (*Revolution*, Spring 1994). Gordon con-

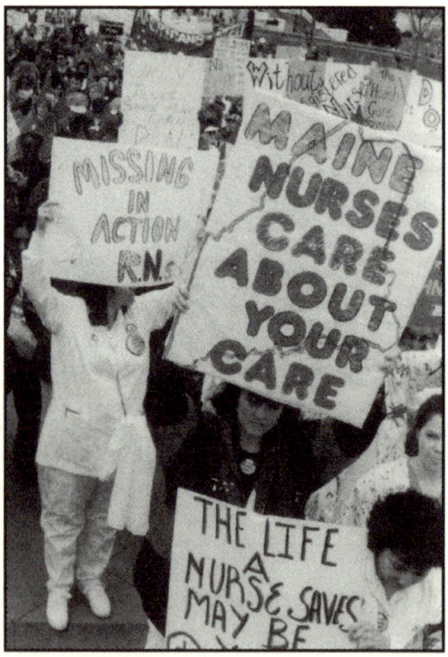
MISSING IN ACTION R.N.
MAINE NURSES CARE ABOUT YOUR CARE
THE LIFE A NURSE SAVES MAY BE

Nurses March on Washington, March 1995. Realizing the calamities facing their profession, nurses took their concerns to the Capitol. (Photo by Mikkel Aaland.)

tinued in this vein: "...hospitals are empty shells to be bought and sold so executives and wealthy stockholders can make a killing."

Corporate America pays little attention to nurses, seeing us as expendable entities whose work can be done more cheaply by someone else. In what can only be seen as a formidable dance of power, there are designated big-time winners and big-time losers. Hospitals, insurance companies, drug companies place themselves in the winner's circle, while nurses, patients, and even some physicians become the sacrificial lambs of the ever popular "patient-focused care."

Since nurses comprise a significant bulk of the work force, we are the first to go. Consultants see numbers and the urge to cut and slash becomes irresistible. After all, these aren't people, just numbers. Nurses are now slated to become "case managers." We get the job done by giving directions, just like traffic cops. Who are we directing? Good question. There are several series of initials that come to mind: PCA, CTA, RCA. These are unlicensed assistive personnel of varying sorts and qualifications, trained for six months, six weeks, six days, or six minutes. These will be the ones in whom families will entrust the care of loved ones.

Take note of the following scenario: A woman in her mid-seventies passes out at home. Her husband calls 911, and she is rushed to the hospital with a blood pressure of 40/20 and dropping. She makes the trip and is settled into the Coronary Care Unit. The nurse who is assigned to this woman reviews the chart and approaches her.

"I see you've lost 30 pounds over the last year," the nurse begins.

"Yes," the patient acknowledges.

"Was your weight loss intentional and monitored by your doctor?"

"Yes."

"Did your doctor make any adjustment in your blood pressure medication to accommodate the change in your weight?" pursues the nurse.

"No," replies the patient.

"I'll make a note to bring this discrepancy to your doctor's attention," says the nurse.

The nurse discusses the matter with the doctor who is understandably embarrassed. An adjustment is made in the medication and the woman goes home a few days later.

It is doubtful that the kind of knowledge displayed by that nurse could be at the fingertips of any of the three initialed wonders. It is also difficult to understand how a nurse who is serving in the capacity of a hall monitor would ever have the opportunity to pick up such a problem.

System, System—Who's Got a System?

Any system that emphasizes saving money is bound to have an adverse effect on just about everyone except those who are advocating the system. In managed competition, the insurance companies are the big winners. In managed care, primary care physicians and insurance companies are the winners. In the single-payer system, the patient appears to be the winner. Where are nurses in all this? Welcome to the "Church of What's Happening Now!"

In California and Massachusetts where managed care has insidiously become a way of life for the medical profession, the effect of this system on nurses was gradual and subtle. In operating rooms and ambulatory surgery centers, for example, caseloads dropped off significantly as specialists realized fewer and fewer referrals. Primary care physicians opt to treat patients themselves, rather than send them to specialists if they can avoid this. For nurses who worked in the OR, PACU, and pre-operative areas, this translated into shorter days and, frequently, unanticipated days off without pay, depending on the prevailing administrative philosophy. On medical-surgical wards, fewer surgeries meant fewer inpatients and involuntary vacation days. Suddenly, we nurses found ourselves scrambling to get in our hours. In a profession notorious for its abundant positions and renowned job security, this status of desperation was shocking and unreal. Yet this was and is the prevailing condition.

In addition, nurses are being laid off in droves. In Massachusetts, 1500 nurses were laid off within a year. Not only are such drastic reductions detrimental to patient care, but it is also absurd to regard nurses as salary-devouring employees, whose termination will bail out a facility anticipating financial catastrophe. Consider this: “In the 1980s, taking inflation into account, RN wages increased a total of 13 percent...In that same period, hospital executive compensation increased by 123 to 142 percent” (*California Nurse,* June 1994, p. 4). Now isn’t that a dazzling and reassuring statistic?!

Ironically, while an article in one section of the newspaper declares that nurses are having no problem getting jobs and at higher salaries, the classifieds for positions for RNs are dwindling, while those for LVNs and Certified Nursing Assistants (CNA) abound. For RNs, this is jarring and requires mental re-grouping to determine where to go from here.

Hey, Hey ANA...Who's Gonna Lay Me Off Today?

As noted earlier, the American Nurses Association has developed the *Nursing's Agenda for Health Care Reform.* The ANA's *Agenda* provides an ordered guideline that might be considered political babble. Nevertheless, it acknowledges that these are chaotic and difficult times for nurses and the *Agenda* attempts to address this matter.

Agenda advocates attest that difficult situations can be avoided when nurses help plan the restructuring. "Nurses' involvement may make the difference between a well-planned restructuring that benefits patients, nurses, and the hospitals alike, and an ill-conceived cost-cutting effort that fails to recognize the realities of our ever-changing environment," notes Elizabeth Farley, vice president of nursing and behavioral health at Saint John's Hospital and Health Care in Santa Monica, California.

Farley points out that at her hospital "cross training, skill-mix changes, and some reduction in work hours per patient day," have allowed savings close to $200,000 a year per med-surg unit, with only a slight reduction in nurse-patient ratios." To further bolster the argument that nurses should actively participate in the restructuring plans at their respective facilities, Farley states that at her hospital no nurse lost her job and that "nurses at the bedside didn't just survive...they benefited." As staff members were cross-trained, nurses were able to do the tasks they were most capable of: assessing the patients individually, "teaching and counseling them, discharge planning, and consulting with caregivers in other disciplines."

As expected, the *Agenda* is controversial and not necessarily embraced enthusiastically by everyone. Critics see the document as a compromise, a corroboration of the "de-skilling" of nursing. In this light, it might also be regarded as the selling out of nursing, for it follows the philosophy that has been nursing's standard: do your job and don't make waves. So what if we're getting farther and farther from the bedside? So what if those assigned to patient care have marginal skills? The important thing is to throw our support with the mainstream ideal and do our best. It is felt that by being a part of the "restructuring" process and working with administrators, nurses will be playing a key role in helping hospitals to survive this period of fiscal uncertainty. Differences in philosophy are one issue. However, with the "de-skilling" of nursing, there is ethical conflict as well as potential legal repercussions (such as lawsuits).

When patient care comes down to "a choice of bad care or no care," notes Julie Pinkham, the associate director of labor relations for the Massachusetts Nurses Association, "It's cause for major concern among nurses." The nurse who comes to work and assesses the situation only to realize that the personnel resources are insufficient (either inadequately trained for the job at hand, or skimpy in number), faces an unpleasant, if not gut-wrenching dilemma: If she refuses to go ahead with the resources allowed, she can be accused of patient abandonment or insubordination; or she can muddle through and hope no incidents occur that could provoke a lawsuit.

Leaders and members of state nursing associations, particularly those in California and Massachusetts where managed care is a way of life, are adamant that restructuring is hazardous to the well-being of patients. The contention is that consultants who are called in to aid in the restructuring process are using an assembly line mentality that may have worked in other industries or businesses, but is totally inappropriate for health care. "We're not talking about automobiles, we're talking about human beings—if you make a mistake on the patient assembly line, you can't recall the product," states Chuck Idelson of the California Nurses Association.

The "fast food" approach to patient care just doesn't work, the restructuring critics assert. The instant satisfaction quotient that has become synonymous with the current American lifestyle will only alienate patients from the knowledge of what is being done to them and for them. One of the ironies of the current health care situation is this: At a period of acute consumer awareness, when patients want another opinion and detailed explanations, the "McDonaldization" of their care precludes their further knowledge and participation.

The subtitle of this chapter asks: "Are We Losing Ground?" The answer is a complex one that cannot be satisfied with a simple "Yes" or "No."

At first glance, the restructuring predicament makes it seem that nurses are losing ground as the threat of mediocre patient care becomes a norm set forth by the high-finance elves. Yet, it is this very dilemma that is allowing us to say "No, we're not losing ground!" Rather, we are gaining momentum each day as the health care debacle compels us to take stock of our situation. For some, the door to unemployment becomes the door to explore new options. For others, restructuring has become a catalyst for action and unification. Threatened by uncertain times, nurses are responding by using the tools of feminism to learn from a movement that seemed to ignore and, in some instances, condemn nurses.

CHAPTER EIGHT

Gloria Steinem, R.N.(!?): Did Feminism Forget Nurses?

Where are We Now?

This chapter is not deliberately contrived to ignore male nurses. Rather, it's an attempt to come to grips with the obvious: nursing has always been, and continues to be, a woman's profession. Granted, more and more men are joining the ranks. Nevertheless, they remain very much a minority and are compelled to face the problems of a "woman's profession:" inadequate salaries for the work involved, overwork/understaffing, verbal (and physical) abuse, and lack of independence.

In the early seventies, when the women's movement was garnering strength and momentum, it was a push for the entire gender. The movement never seemed to fracture itself into special interests: teachers, secretaries, physicians, engineers, nurses, astronauts. The idea was that, as the gender found itself and staked its claims, those in diverse careers would realize the rewards of the gender battle. In truth, this happened. In nursing it just didn't happen enough.

In 1990, Betty Freidan, who was and continues to be at the forefront of the women's movement, acknowledged that feminism had become bogged down. Feminist proponents were aware and well versed in the problems facing women, but they had failed to move forward to alter the significant areas of power: government and the workplace.

In the latter, nursing and feminism are in tandem. In fact, nursing may even be a bit ahead in this tedious struggle for equality, where progress is measured in millimeters rather than fifty yard gains (no field goals or touchdowns, here!).

Nurses, too, recognize the problems inherent in their profession. Let's face it, how can you be a nurse and **not** be aware of the problems. However, alterations at the powerbase are rare. It is here that the similarities between the factions of nursing and feminism end. In many ways, it would seem that nursing and the women's movement are suffering from irreconcilable differences. However, there is hope.

Feminism and Nursing: What Went Wrong?

Why did feminism ignore nursing? The women's movement chose to eschew professions that adhered to traditional women's roles. In its efforts to propel women to equality and recognition, the movement urged women to look at those vocations previously dominated by men. The world is our oyster, too, declared the movement. There is no reason why women can't become doctors, lawyers, senators, bankers, and candlestick makers. In the momentum to press forward, nursing, as a "woman's profession," was cast aside and regarded by many with a jaundiced eye.

Nursing embodied everything that the women's movement was trying to overcome: an oppressed profession with a long-standing history of dealing with a condescending patriarchy, overwork, underpay, and elements of physical and verbal abuse thrown in for good measure. You would think that the profession was made-to-order for a total feminist overhaul. But this was not the case. Nursing was seen as an embarrassment. "Go away. Nursing is hopeless," opined the feminist hierarchy. "Nursing is everything we're trying to forget."

Logic dictates that feminism and nursing should be cohorts, bravely locking arms to fight the battles that beset womanhood. This is a valid conclusion, in theory. Unhappily, the reality is less positive, as Ellen Baer states in "The Feminist Disdain for Nursing:" "...the terrible paradox of feminism [is that it] glorifies women who emulate masculine behavior while virtually ignoring women who choose traditionally female roles and careers... feminism... abandons feminine caring roles in order to achieve progress" (*The New York Times*, February 23, 1991, p. 24). To gain equality in the world of men, it is better for a woman to be a doctor than a nurse. Accordingly, it only follows that in 1986 enrollment of women in medical schools surpassed that of women in nursing schools. To be in a traditional "woman's profession" apparently undermined the tenets of the feminist movement.

Yet, if you take a close look at the plight of nurses, you can more easily understand the plight of women in general. Baer stresses the importance of feminists to recognize and "...address the needs of women doing women's work." If feminism is to succeed for all women, it isn't enough for women to have equal access to all fields. It is essential that "traditionally female professions like nursing gain the high value and solid social respect they deserve" (Baer, p. 24).

It should be the mutual goal of both feminists and nurses to make nursing an attractive profession. It should be a career that offers divergent paths, improved status, high self-esteem, decent wages, and autonomy. The profession should be one that encourages creativity and innovation. Nurses' efforts to make improvements in patient care (not to mention cost-effectiveness!) need to be acknowledged and rewarded.

Nursing and Feminism: Righting the Wrong

While feminists have displayed a disdain for nursing as a "woman's profession," the true irony is that, in order to progress past the image and reality of an oppressed group, nurses must look to the strengths of feminism.

In her book, *Nursing and Health Care*, author Peggy Chinn states that "Feminism is much more than a slogan. It is a profound insight about the world that creates a tremendous shift in how we think, what we identify as the most important problems in our world today and what solutions we envision for these problems." Chinn continues by asserting, "This insight brings us face to face with issues of power and freedom... what it means to be powerful and what it means to exercise power in the world."

Power and freedom do not come easily. They are not handed out as samples at the supermarket and they can't be bought with Visa or Mastercard. To enjoy power and freedom, nurses must come to grips with and conquer several obstacles.

The first major hurdle that we nurses face as individuals and as a group is learning to believe in ourselves. It would be great if such a belief could be taught or offered in a continuing education seminar. But it isn't. So what do we do? We look at our skills and take an inventory of what we do at work each day. How many IVs did we start? How many patients (and their families) were comforted by what we said and information we provided? Take a look at all the equipment that requires our knowledge—microscopes, power equipment, monitors, machines that go "Beep" in the night. Underneath the surface, we nurses **know** that we are good at what we do. If we didn't believe in our talents and skills, we couldn't go to work each day, we couldn't care for our patients.

Caring is not unique to nursing alone. It is also an abiding feminist ethic. However, as noted in their article "Power at the Policy Table—When Women and Nurses are Involved," (*Revolution*, Summer 1993), Barbara Backer et al point out that caring is really not gender specific. "It is a value that *must* be central to the foundations, operations and priorities of the workplace, government, organizations and the community." The authors continue: "Caring involves a belief system that encourages empowerment and emancipation of both nurses and patients. It encompasses fostering a health care system that is comprised of enabling and supportive activities."

It has been noted by many astute observers that nurses have long been working in a society that does not truly value caring. Working in such a society has created a conflict for nurses and has taken its toll on the profession. Becker and her associates observe: "It has led men to view nursing as an inappropriate profession for them (although this may be changing as wages for nurses increase and availability of traditional, male-dominated jobs decreases) and, more recently, for many women to view it disparagingly."

Despite the indifferent view of society towards the art of caring, we nurses (men and women) have rediscovered and renewed our commitment to caring—for ourselves and for our patients. This renewal has led to the first tenuous step for nurses to unite and speak out on behalf of our commitment.

Since we are knowledgeable, our voices should be heard. After all, we are experienced and smart—and we care.

Self-esteem and Empowerment: We Have to Start Someplace

Empowerment, which began in the late '80s, is really where feminism and nursing meet. For nurses, it means shoring ourselves up as individuals and as a profession. In the article, "Toward a Feminist Model for the Political Empowerment of Nurses" (*Revolution*, Spring 1993), the authors define empowerment as "the enabling of people and groups of people to act and make decisions where an equitable distribution of power exists."

For nurses, this means:

- Balancing out the unequal sociopolitical scales that hamper our profession
- Developing and maintaining positive self-esteem
- Generating the necessary political skills to deal with and give input to the changes in the health care system

The phrase "balancing out the unequal sociopolitical scales" is nice and ambiguous. What the term really means is that as nurses, we must make our place one that is recognized and respected by our counterparts in the medical world.

The inequalities experienced in nursing mirror those in mainstream society: racial, ethnic, and class prejudices. However, these are not the only problems we face. We are also bogged down by nurses who hang on to outdated views which stipulate that any sort of political behavior, interest, or activity is neither feminine nor professional. So what do we do to correct this? We employ integration. This sort of integration does not require marching through the South singing *We Shall Overcome*. It is more of an internal tool.

Integration allows one to work within the system by determining and valuing one's own perspective and opinion. "This [valuing one's own perspective and opinion] is evident in nursing's public and professional reaffirmation of caring as its essence in the face of exploding technology and society's expectations of cure," says writer Virginia Sapiro (*Revolution*, Spring 1993). Integration is vital if a profession is to realize changes in its power structure, values, and priorities.

For nurses, integration means that we value our perspectives and ourselves as men and women. It's time to use the "S" word again—**self-esteem**!

> We must take responsibility for our happiness and stop blaming and directing control outside of ourselves. Grab hold of all that you are. Discover new and different aspects of yourself and life—Through a happy, positive set of glasses—They are there, waiting for you to put them on.
>
> —*Helene Nawrocki, RN, MSN*

Aren't you tired of hearing how oppressed we nurses are? Aren't you sick of looking for your self-esteem under chairs and under beds? Well, it's time to stop sniveling and get with the program! It's time to come to grips with who and what we are. Enter empowerment!

To develop and raise our self-esteem is a chore that must come from within each of us. We must acknowledge our talents and promote ourselves accordingly. Additionally, it is our task to educate the public. This is especially tough when an author like Robin Norwood, comments in her book, *Women Who Love Too Much*, that women from dysfunctional families are "over represented" in fields like nursing. In 1988, *Working Woman* magazine listed nursing in its report on the "Ten Worst Jobs." We definitely have our work cut out for us!

It is also frustrating to find that those who are allegedly on our side are sniping at us in guerrilla war fashion with statements like Luther Christman made in "The Future of the Nursing Profession" (*Nursing Administration Quarterly*, Winter 1987): "A certain aura of anti-intellectualism has always been apparent within the (nursing) profession." Shall we throw ourselves under a train because we lack an interest in Sartre or Plato? Should country music lovers be condemned because they fail to lust for the strains of a Wagnerian opera? Does this mean that our expertise in advanced cardiac life support is nullified by our inability to differentiate between the works of Monet and Van Gogh?

It has long been my contention that what separates nurses and doctors is that we've read different books, taken different tests, and passed different boards. We are as bright (if not brighter) than those who cast such long shadows. Empowerment is the acknowledgment of this. It also calls for nurses to pull together as a group, which is finally occurring albeit very slowly. Yet mutual respect can be the necessary component here. A feminist model for empowerment calls for "political action [which] includes respect for others and for self, power-sharing and equality" (*Revolution*, Spring 1993).

This "political action" manifests itself keenly in the "development of a sense of injustice." It is one thing to tolerate injustice and resign oneself to it; but it is an altogether different matter to recognize injustice and take action to right the wrong when possible. Nurses are in a tough position. For so many of the difficult situations we face are part and parcel of the systems in which we work and, as such, the problems cannot be remedied quickly or easily by action of any sort. To create changes of the magnitude required to revamp the ancient systems entrenched in the medical community is an awesome task, indeed. Yet, it is not impossible. Changes can come about by picking away at the small timbers that make up the foundations. It requires a steady and dedicated tenacity, which might be as effortless as offering alternative solutions to proposed plans or subtlely questioning a rule or guideline that might be outdated or unreasonable.

As the self-esteem of individual nurses increases, the profession itself will ultimately realize a transformation. This is becoming evident as "restructuring" eliminates traditional nursing roles in hospitals; forcing us to revamp our career paths and make choices that were previously seen as impractical and impossible. In addition, our voices are being heard throughout the country as nurses speak out against the compromising of patient care in the wake of "restructuring."

Takin' It to the Streets

In an effort to find our collective voice and to have that voice heard, registered nurses are learning that while loud is good, public is better. As a means of protest, we are literally taking to the streets to air our complaints and to educate the public.

> There is nothing I love as much as a good fight.
>
> —*Franklin Delano Roosevelt*

The Nurses March on Washington, which took place in the nation's capitol on March 31, 1995, is perhaps the strongest example. The event attracted media attention and put the consumer on notice that, due to massive RN layoffs and the hiring of questionably qualified personnel, patient care in hospitals is being compromised in an unprecedented manner. The voices were unified, loud, strong, clear, and the message left nothing to misinterpretation: **Budgets Slashed; Patients Trashed.**

Across the nation, nurses are protesting intolerable situations:

- ➢ At Carney Hospital in Boston, staffing "adjustments" were put on hold after widespread RN protests.
- ➢ In 1994, in Stockton California, the RNs at St. Joseph's Medical Center filed a charge of unfair labor practices to protest the newly implemented team concept, which nurses felt undermined the care patients received.

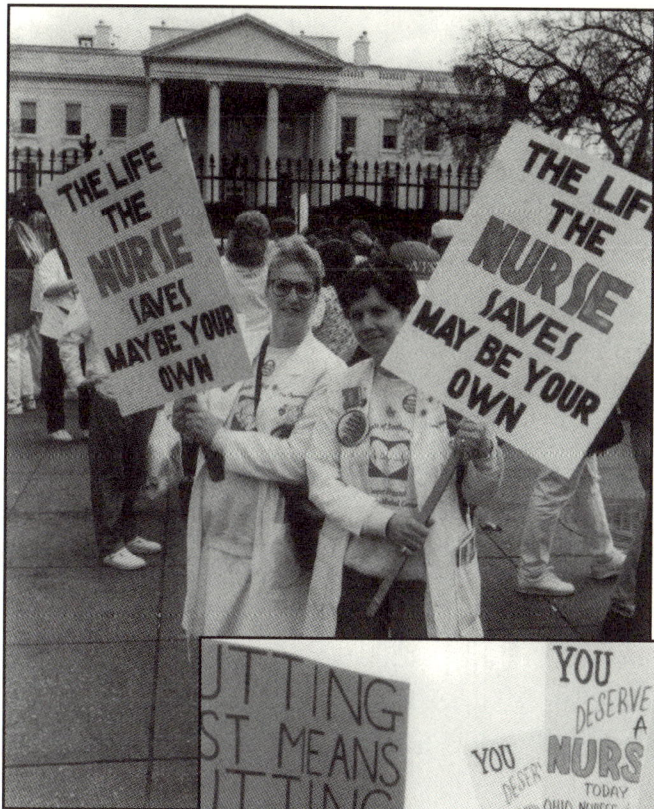

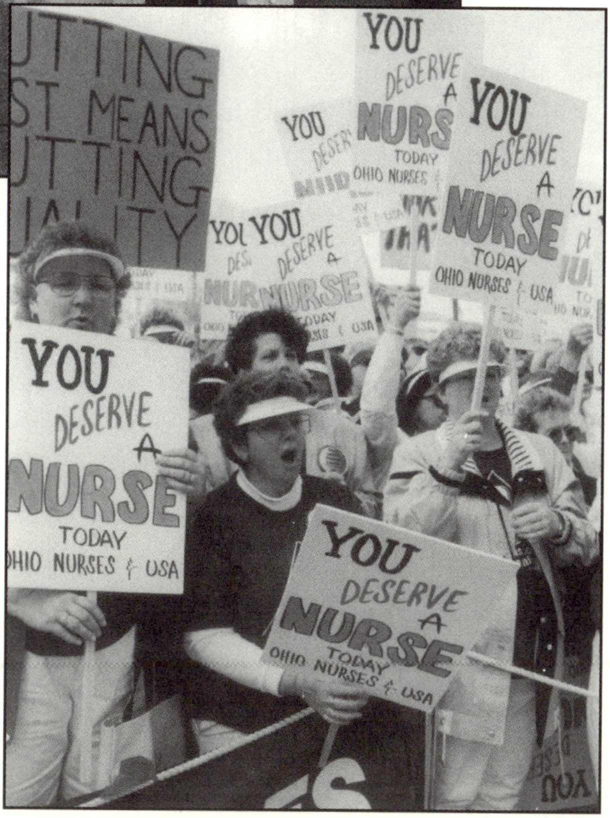

Nurses March on Washington, March 31, 1995. (Photos:Mikkel Aaland.)

- A peaceful rally was held in San Francisco in May 1994. More than 300 RNs and their supporters marched for "quality care and quality jobs." This served as a means not only to vent anger and frustration caused by "restructuring," but also it was a method to educate the public to the perils it faces as quality of health care is sacrificed.

- Early in 1995, Alta Bates Medical Center in Berkeley, California established two pilot units to test the idea of "restructuring." More than 80 percent of those who staffed the units signed petitions wherein they refused to "act as supervisors" of unlicensed "care associates" who would replace some of the nurses. The California Nurses Association held a press conference outside the hospital and charged that the pilot units endangered patients' safety.

- The American Nurses Association, in the spring of 1995, launched a national drive to alert and, hopefully, convince the public that "Every Patient Deserves a Nurse." The ANA got the word out through distribution of more than 50,000 brochures, newspapers, and public service announcements.

- In Port Jervis, New York, nurses at Mercy Community Hospital staged a hunger strike to protest the hospital breaking off negotiations with nurses and hiring replacements. This move by the hospital was condemned by Cardinal John O'Conner and by Bishop Tom Gumbleton of Detroit, where Mercy Health Services is headquartered.

- In January 1995, the Illinois Nurses Association claimed a decisive victory in its negotiations with the University of Illinois Hospital. More than 90% of the nurses employed at the hospital ratified a contract which allowed for a 3.5% pay raise. The agreement was regarded as a major victory to overturn the facility's plan to replace RNs with technicians and unlicensed assistive personnel. In addition, the pact called for guaranteed nursing positions and the involvement of nurses in budget-setting, stiffened layoff criteria, and stipulated nurses' rights to make decisions through delegation. It also emphasized that staff nurses wouldn't be considered supervisors simply because they delegated responsibilities to lesser-skilled workers.

Citizens in the Land of the Dollar Bill

In the late 1980s, the *Washington Post* reported that hospital maintenance workers were earning more money than registered nurses. A study in Illinois concluded that electricians were commanding annual salaries close to $9,000 more than nurses. In 1988, nurses in Maine were driving to Massachusetts on weekends because two Saturday and Sunday shifts allowed them to bring home more money that a full week's work in their home state. When hundreds of state-employed nurses threatened to resign from Denver University Hospital rather than accept a salary freeze, they were joined by other nurses and supported by physicians, and hospital administrators (God must live in Colorado!). Legislators ultimately relented.

Kaiser, the largest HMO in California, constantly claims to be in the throes of a financial crisis. Newspapers are filled with stories of building projects being put on hold or possibly abandoned. Talks of nursing layoffs abound and administration and management positions in several facilities have been restructured to eliminate and combine different jobs. In 1994, at one of its facilities, Kaiser requested that 23 benefited RNs voluntarily leave. The "severance package" touted was a week's pay and medical/dental coverage for each year of "benefited" service with the HMO. Seniority offered a dubious cushion, but a cushion nonetheless. If more than 23 nurses opted to leave, only those with the most seniority would receive a benefits package. If less than 23 nurses volunteered to go, those with the least seniority would be asked to leave and would receive the severance package.

Despite all of this hand-wringing and frantic posturing, in July 1994, the physicians in this HMO received a letter informing them that their incomes would be increased in light of stable financial conditions that prevailed. To wit: "we are meeting our financial targets." There must have been an accounting miracle to which only the medical staff was privy!

Nurses will not dispute that salaries have improved. But how good is the money? At first glance, nurses' salaries look fairly decent. We have seen our wages increase and this in itself is progress. Nevertheless, this financial advance is somewhat deceptive.

Figures provided by the Bureau of Labor Statistics reveal that during the ten-year period from 1983-1993, the median weekly earnings for registered nurses increased from $411 to $687. This reflects change of 40%. For physicians, the change is more dramatic. Their median weekly earnings virtually doubled from $502 in 1983 to $1,019 in 1993. (It should be emphasized that these figures represent a mean for all physicians: from the plastic surgeon to the stars in Beverly Hills to the rural general practitioner in East Belt Buckle, Tennessee.)

Now for the good news: Managed care may prove to be the great financial equalizer. Already, in areas where managed care has a foothold (some would say a stranglehold), physicians are seeing 35%-40% drops in their incomes. Meanwhile, RNs are gearing up for change by becoming nurse practitioners and physician assistants, along with other more lucrative careers within their discipline. These changes call for increased salaries as well as increased responsibilities. It is still not recommended that one choose nursing as a means to become a millionaire! Nevertheless, it can be expected that the financial gap between doctors and nurses will be reduced.

Standing Up for Ourselves at Last

As we strive to unload the baggage of submissiveness, sexist perceptions, and deferential behavior, we nurses are consciously working to alter our image of ourselves. It is not immoral to put ourselves first and further our own interests. New role models, assertive, intellectual men and women who realize their potential, are needed at the forefront of health care.

There is growing evidence that this positive image is becoming an actuality. In January 1993, 350 nurses out of a bargaining unit of 630 at St. Joseph's Hospital in Peoria, Illinois went on strike. The key issues for the nurses were "quality of patient care, professional respect and a fair contract" ("Strike!" by Dawn Chipman, *Revolution*, Winter 1993). The nurses had enough of being farmed out to work in areas in which they were unfamiliar and unskilled. They were tired of beating their heads against the administration wall that regarded them as whiners and complainers. One involved RN observed: "...when nurses get fed up enough to fight for what they want, change does happen."

In Kentucky, when legislators tried to add a new tax to nurses' salaries based on a new federal regulation "that adds 'nurses' services' to the list of providers and services that states can choose to tax to finance their match for Medicaid dollars" (*AJN*, January 1994), the folks in the state capitol got a rude awakening. After a searing letter-writing campaign, prompted by the Kentucky Nurses Association, which elicited a deluge of thousands of letters, state officials backed off. Their stand was corroborated by the Health Care Financing Administration that stated the rule was never meant to apply "to individual nurses' pay."

Nurses in Alabama won a victory in February 1994 when a court decision stipulated that the Alabama State Committee of Public Health had exceeded its statutory authority by proposing that ED (emergency department) paramedics were to provide nursing services (*AJN*, June 1994). A coalition of nurses, supported financially by the Emergency Nurses Association, filed the successful suit.

In case we can't handle current challenges ourselves, we can always rely on the federal government for assistance(?!). Recently, Congress authorized the federal Institute of Medicine to "explore the relationship between nurse staffing levels, patient care and workplace injuries suffered by nurses. At a cost of $900,000, the new commission is charged with solving problems created by health care employers who followed the recommendations of the first national commission in 1989" (*Modern Healthcare*, July 18, 1994). It was the recommendation of the first commission that non-nursing duties (secretarial, janitorial, the usual tasks nurses do because there is no one else to do them) be reassigned to non-nursing personnel. This was a follow-up to the commission's findings that the nursing shortage was caused by hospitals hiring too many nurses who were doing too many non-nursing jobs. If it sounds confusing, it is! The government has a knack for making the simple complicated and duplicating the effort.

Are We Mouthy or Courageous?

For nurses, the climb out of oppression is an uneven one, a dance of two steps forward, one step back. When we try to stand up for ourselves, point out problems in our departments, request attention to errors and mismanagement, we're labeled "troublemakers." The Supreme Court has presented itself as an especially menacing foe in two decisions it recently handed down.

In one instance, a nurse was fired for insubordination by a hospital when she complained about the working conditions in her department and this was reported to her supervisor. The main opinion set forth by Justice Sandra Day O'Connor stated that "employees can be fired for making insubordinate statements even if they made other statements that would be constitutionally protected free speech" and that the employer uses "the care that a reasonable manager would use before making an employment decision" (*The Sacramento Bee*, June 1, 1994, p. F1). Essentially what this means is that "an employer cannot be held liable to firing someone who it believed made statements unprotected by free speech." While the decision set aside the ruling by the appellate court, it nevertheless allowed the lawsuit to go forward.

In another ruling, the Court stipulated that "nurses who direct the work of other employees could potentially be deemed supervisors under the federal labor law, and thus deprived of collective bargaining rights and workplace protections" (*California Nurse*, June 1994). In the past, "the National Labor Relations Board has held that a nurse is not considered a supervisor when directing co-workers as part of her professional duties."

The aforementioned Court decision comes at a time that is critical for nurses. As "restructuring" takes hold, we nurses will find ourselves responsible for the actions of non-RNs. Indeed, it can be anticipated that "employers will step up efforts to place registered nurses in situations that give the appearance of supervisory status." This will become particularly poignant when contracts are up for renewal and hospitals challenge the status of RNs in this supervisory capacity. Membership in bargaining units will require definitive clarification. While efforts are underway to have this ruling overturned, this matter emphasizes the difficulties nurses can expect in the future.

Each generation of nurses brings the profession a little closer to modern life and modern philosophy, be it feminism, tolerance, equality, or assertiveness. Many of these attributes are developed in nursing school. Nursing schools have the significant responsibility of providing graduates with the wherewithal to survive and improve the lot of their chosen profession.

Each decade, bright, fresh-faced graduates enter hospitals armed with new ideals and values. In the 1960s, student nurses were taught to relinquish their chairs to physicians who came to the nurses' station. I don't think that's part of the curriculum today. The students of the 1990s do not intend to relinquish anything.

CHAPTER NINE

Nursing Schools and Education

Let's Start at the Very Beginning

The tone was set in nursing school. It was there that the nurses' worst enemy was born and cultivated. It was an insidious foe, bred from within and fostered from without. Indeed, our greatest adversary was our own self-image.

In the past, nursing programs isolated their students, usually through the frantic adage: too much to learn, too little time. Faculties in such programs sought to mold their haplessly eager charges into their own image. Nursing instructors were clichés: unmarried women who inadvertently transferred their own misery onto their students. Fear was their modus operandi and they wielded their power with relentless vengeance, all under the guise of dedication and camaraderie. As student nurses, we were trained, rather than educated. We were military recruits, privates in the army of medicine where conformity was gospel and our unquestioning servitude in this patriarchal world was essential to survival.

Self-esteem was stifled and we were taught blind obedience and unflagging loyalty. Independent thought was squelched. The emphasis on nursing was total and complete with little or no opportunity to explore eclectic pursuits. Even those of us participating in a community college program that required non-nursing courses as part of a basic curriculum were confined to the basics: English, American history, political science. No opportunity was allowed the student to dabble in a literature or an art history course. Those of us who were enrolled in nursing programs in two-year colleges were reminded that we were different. We were unique. We were nurses.

My classmates and I were a motley group. We were caught up in our own mystique that was tempered by our naiveté. Our uniforms set us apart from the rest of the student body at the community college. The lab coats we wore during microbiology distinguished us at break time when we gathered around the flagpole to flaunt our uniqueness to the world and smoke cigarettes (yes, I went to school a *long* time ago!).

Yet, we were also aware of the gravity of our course of study. Once past the bed baths and into the throes of pharmacology, our learning took on the aspect of fear. Nowhere was it more apparent how critical our roles were than with the administration of medications. Any omission or inaccurate dosage could be dangerous at best, fatal at worst.

The idea of being a patient advocate, per se, was never vocalized. Tenderness and caring were ingrained in the profession, but then so was obsequiousness. The doctor was the Wizard of Oz, a deity of sorts, seemingly infallible. His word was the final decree, never to be questioned.

As students, we were the lowest beings on medicine's professional totem pole. It was our duty to absorb the knowledge that was thrown our way, devour it and regurgitate it at the appropriate moment. We were the children of the medical world, there to be seen and not heard. After two years, we were beige entities, able to blend into any and all backgrounds, content to go about our business without question. We were dedicated and we were martyrs, not an unusual combination.

Yet, we were the lucky ones. We got our wake up call early on in the '60s and '70s. For those nurses who were older and "more experienced," the brainwashing of nursing school could not be erased. They were locked into an old philosophy and they were reluctant to part with the overriding tenor of a philosophy so deeply ingrained. What happened?

A combination of events occurred. Throughout the nation, people were taking a stand and making their voices heard. From feminists to malcontented, disillusioned students defending freedom of speech, fighting for women's rights, and demonstrating against the Vietnam war, people were protesting and fighting back.

By comparison, nurses made quiet strides. Any attempt to move forward (salary increases, retirement benefits) was regarded by the general public as disgraceful and devoid of dedication, especially if it involved a strike. Nurses waged their war in whispers. To do otherwise countered a tradition of subservience; it defied the teachings held so dear in nursing school. It took nurses a long time to heed the call for change.

Nursing schools, while initially slow to respond to the modifications in nursing, have, for the most part, risen from their slumber. Nursing educators realize that they must not only change, but must also lead the way to change—the change toward empowerment.

Heading Toward the 21st Century

Empowerment is a critical component of the nursing education process. It is a positive element that provides a student with the necessary tools to succeed in today's wild medical climate. By learning to be leaders, critical thinkers and problem solvers, nursing students can approach their discipline with a sense of collegiality, self-respect, and professionalism. There is no room for mechanical thinking and passivity in nursing. Ours is a profession that is pro-active, not re-active.

How do nursing schools and nursing educators go about the task of producing a nurse who will survive "out there?" The ruling powers of nursing programs who determine the curriculum, hire the instructors, and admit the students must realize the importance of coordinating these three elements. It is the integration of these three components that creates the empowered nurse.

The Curriculum

Much of the curriculum of a nursing program is standard. Students still must learn the basics of care: giving bed baths, taking vital signs, charting patient care, administering medications. Yet courses should also be eclectic. It is essential that college graduates be more than one-dimensional, although there is no doubt that nursing is an exacting discipline. Happily, nursing education is becoming quite varied. It has taken a while, but the world is finally recognizing that nurses are more than cute white caps and sensible shoes. Nurses are smart and possess a curiosity about their entire world, beyond the hospital. Accordingly, time is being allotted for the wonderful variety of knowledge offered through liberal arts classes. The perspectives of Plato, James Joyce, and Francis Bacon are relevant in every field. Aristotle said that "education is the best provision for old age." It is also the best tool for nurses. The more one knows, the better equipped one is to do a good job.

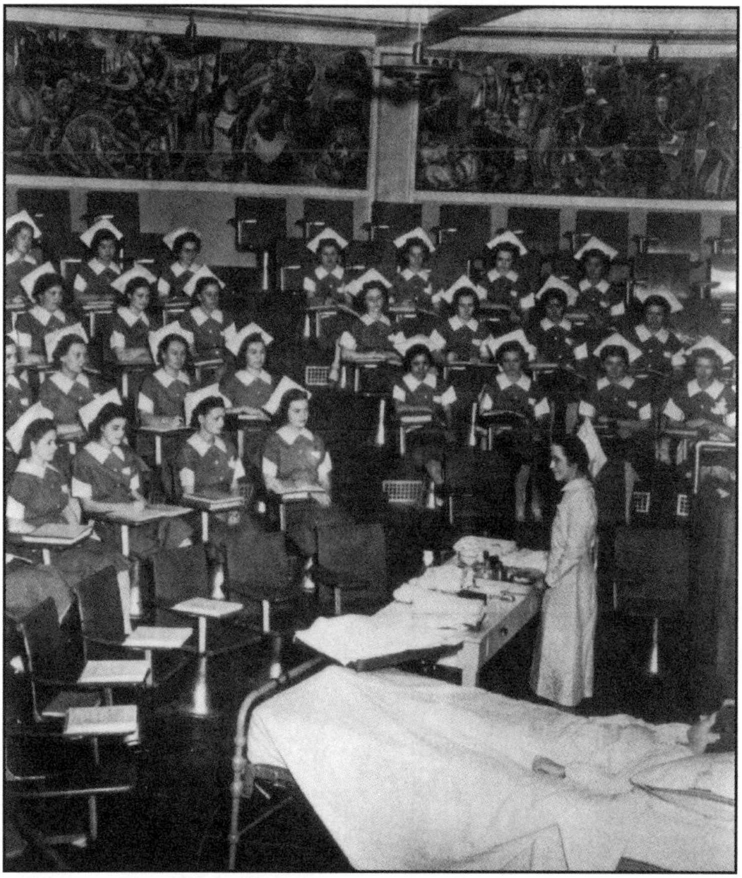

Student nurses in class at University of California San Francisco c. 1948. (Courtesy UCSF archives.)

As alternatives to hospital nursing become the rule, rather than the exception, nursing schools are broaching the subject of these alternatives in their curricula.

A nationwide inquiry was conducted for this book to see how nursing schools were preparing their students for the changes they will face in the brave new world of health care. The responses received show that educators are no longer shying away from the innovative. Courses offered are varied and timely and allow students the opportunity to explore.

Required upper division courses at Cailfornia State University, Sacramento (a program that confers a Bachelor of Science degree in Nursing at graduation) are: Bridging Constructs for Returning Nurses, Leadership and Management in Nursing Practice, Community Health Nursing, Research in Nursing. Among the courses that nurses might choose to fulfill an additional graduation requirement are Health Care: Issues and Delivery Systems, Women's Health, Culture and Poverty, Contemporary American Culture, and Human Sexuality.

Macon College, a two-year program in Macon, Georgia, offers a course in Interpersonal Communications as part of the mandatory nursing courses. The concepts of managed care are covered in the first nursing class, Fundamentals of Nursing. As they progress through the program, students are taught about the changes in health care and how these changes will affect them.

A response from Norfolk State University in Virginia revealed that the nursing program increasingly uses the community as a client to provide the Bachelor of Science students opportunities in leadership and management. The school offers courses in Research Dimensions in Nursing, Multiculturalism/Bioethics, Humanities, and African-American Perspectives. Students are also required to take Computer Concepts before they are admitted to the nursing program. The junior year offers the most varied course of study in the four-year program: Colloquium, Statistics, Principles of Economics, or American Public Policy, as well as a free elective and a humanities elective.

The B.S. in Nursing Program at The Jewish Hospital College of Nursing and Allied Health in St. Louis, Missouri, offers a variety of humanities and business courses as part of the non-nursing curriculum. Among the classes offered are Logic, Introduction to Art, Masterpieces in Literature, Introduction to Political Economy, Ethics, Business Organization, and Administration and Supervisory Management. Nursing courses that are required include Research Methods in Nursing, Community Health, Leadership and Management in Nursing.

The examples are fairly representative of what is being offered to students throughout the country. The content of the curricula suggests that those in charge of nursing programs no longer seek to isolate their students with limited fields of study. Program directors and administrators are realizing, at last, that for nurses to be effective, they must have diversity in their education. Other fields of study can contribute to the **whole** nurse, making him or her a valuable asset to any facility.

General nursing courses continue to be the backbone of any nursing program. These courses are also being updated to meet the contemporary demands that nurses continue to face.

Holistic nursing and preventative care are currently being emphasized. Students are experiencing the duties of home health care through unique programs that bring them into neighborhoods. Some of these centers are the creations of the students themselves, staffed by students. Programs that bring students into the community, such as speaking in public schools about AIDS, and working in prenatal clinics that focus on teen mothers, are encouraged. Students are made aware of opportunities in research, utilization review, writing, and nursing in culturally different environments (Indian reservations, working outside the United States). Presenting nursing as the broad spectrum career it is becoming prepares students to enter their chosen field fully aware of all possibilities.

Areas in nursing that require additional education are not overlooked. Students know the additional doors that post-graduate work opens to them—nurse practitioner, physician assistant, Certified Registered Nurse Anesthetist (CRNA), managerial positions.

Nursing students who are well versed in the available options enter their profession with confidence and assurance. They can be forever grateful to their instructors for this preparation and encouragement.

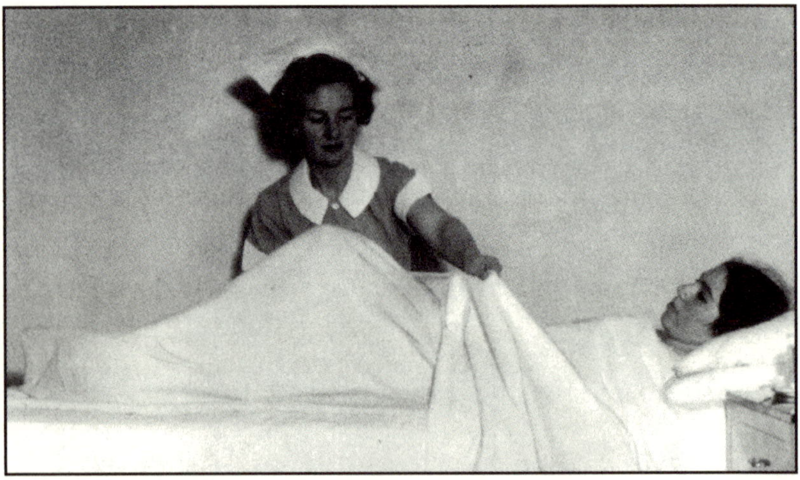

Bed making as part of the fundamentals of nursing at UCSF c. 1950. (Courtesy UCSF archives.)

The Educators

Perhaps the most salient gift a nursing educator can offer students is individuality coupled with enthusiasm. Instructors who approach their areas of expertise in unique and diverse ways will be well remembered as will the content of the courses they teach. It takes a fair degree of courage to stand up for individuality, particularly if nursing program higher-ups are reluctant to change and press for formulaic teaching: "We've been successful with this method for the last 100 years. Why should we change now?"

To keep matters in perspective and to appreciate the progress nursing education has made during the last 25-30 years, let's return, once more, to the Neolithic Age when I went to nursing school. (Giving injections with those needles carved from stone was tough!)

In the hospital setting, nursing students traveled in groups. We were little pods of people who moved through the hospital corridors as a well-starched mass. At the head of our group was our instructor who kept a wary eye on her charges and made certain that no one lagged.

It was embarrassing on one level. We moved about in groups of six or eight, chattering and giggling, well aware of the patients' curiosity and the staff's dread. The image of baby chicks being guided by the mother hen was ever-present. However, our anonymity was obliterated once we received our assignments. Then, removed from the shelter of the group cocoon, we assumed, once more, our individuality and its inherent responsibilities. We were set loose upon unsuspecting, bedridden patients, who had no choice but to endure our trial and error as we honed our budding skills.

Our immediate destiny as nursing students was to be whipped into shape. We were perceived as brainless, senseless and, on occasion, hopeless. No thought was given to building self-esteem, let alone developing the qualities of empowerment. It was the nursing instructor's goal to perpetuate the misery and subservience of the profession.

Such are the facts and lessons of history. Fast forwarding to the present reveals a different picture. On some campuses, there may be vestiges of "the old school." The philosophy of the old guard might still be applied (hopefully only by instructors who are nearing retirement). The prevailing atmosphere not only of medicine, but also of society has compelled nursing education to take a close look at itself and to adapt accordingly.

Nursing education has made significant strides toward introducing the power of positive thinking. Today, instructors are urged to treat students as "professionals-in-training" or "junior colleagues." Hopefully, by encouraging students as valuable newcomers, the properties of self-esteem, leadership, and empowerment will evolve.

It is no longer acceptable to emphasize dependence and blind obedience or, for that matter, the ultimate calamity of the profession: the death of the patient. The possibility of patient demise should be used as a valuable tool to encourage independent thinking and to trust personal observations, rather than as a weapon to instill fear and indecisiveness.

Our educators were not innovative. However, in all fairness, nursing education in 1966 was not creative in an instructional sense. It was not nursing's mission then to be clever and invent new challenges. The discipline itself was thought to be provocative enough.

Change keeps people stimulated and alive. Imagine the dreariness of having to teach the same subject, the same way year after year. There is nothing more disappointing than to take a class (compulsory, no less) that is taught by someone who is dull and mired in the subject matter. In contrast, a class, no matter how difficult, can be irresistible and fascinating when the teacher generates unbridled enthusiasm for the topic.

One of the most difficult classes I had as a student at UC Berkeley was in Japanese history. Yet, the professor had such a love for the subject that it was contagious. I looked forward to my classes each week and studied with great dedication for the killer exams. My grade wasn't the best, but I developed an interest in Japanese history that goes beyond sushi and Sony Walkmans to this day.

Teachers have a duty to instill in their students a pride in their craft as well as self-esteem in their capabilities. It is truly objectionable, in this day and age, for instructors to be mentally abusive to students, to upbraid them and ridicule them in front of their peers. Nursing is tough enough without all that garbage. Patients want the nurse who is caring for them to be confident in his or her skills, independent and creative, as well as protective and caring. Better to have a nurse whose morale and self-respect were encouraged than to be cared for by a nurse who was constantly beaten down and isolated in theories that make stone age wisdom seem avant garde.

More and more, nursing educators are teaching students to be assertive ("tactfully aggressive") for this is the first step toward empowerment. Educators realize the importance of assertiveness and they are incorporating "how to" in their curricula. To be an assertive nurse is more than standing up to administration and physicians when they make questionable decisions. It's also recognizing when change is needed and assuming responsibility for one's actions, whether right or wrong.

Today's nursing students are motivated to be flexible, to be aware of all options and to consider those which are most appropriate. This can be instilled in the classroom where assignments are presented in a variety of forms: written papers, oral presentations, play acting, seminar and group discussions.

There is more to education than memorizing endless facts and figures and spewing them out upon demand. Students must be motivated to think on their feet, to be challenged with real life scenarios. A scanning of the daily newspaper can provide a wealth of situations that might be presented to students under the guise of "What would you do in this situation, based upon what we learned in class yesterday?" A situation such as the bombing of the Federal Building in Oklahoma City can offer vast avenues for "What would you do...?"

- What would priorities be in the emergency room as a staff nurse? As a charge nurse?
- How would you set up a triage system for hundreds of patients coming in with multiple injuries? With single injuries?
- How would you handle the pediatric patients? The adult patients?
- What would you do as an OR nurse in the same situation?
- How would you prepare your ward for multiple arrivals of post-op or ER patients?
- If you were at the scene, how would you go about taking care of people?

The Oklahoma City bombing is, thankfully, a rare experience. However, the daily newspapers are full of stories on a more ordinary level: the family struggling with a young child dying of cancer might warrant a discussion of pediatric cancer treatment, the effects of chemotherapy, the devastation leukemia wreaks on the body, the psychological problems that affect individual family members, etc. The horseback riding accident of actor Christopher Reeve might open the door to reviewing neurosurgical procedures and techniques as well as nursing care of the quadriplegic, rehabilitation, working with the depressed patient. Such a situation might also spark a debate about euthanasia or assisted suicide. Applying textbook information to everyday situations with actual names and faces infuses medicine and nursing care with real people and makes learning easier and more memorable. ("I remember, they did that procedure when that Olympic skier broke her leg." or "We set up a mock triage like that when we read about the World Trade Center bombing in New York City. In fact, we did such and such. Would that be helpful here?")

Practical applications of facts are invaluable. After all, how many of us have called up from the recesses of our minds what we learned in our high school algebra or geometry classes? On the surface, the information force-fed us in these classes seems utterly useless. Yet, the real value is that these courses taught us to think in a certain way, and while the equations have long since dropped off our mental map, the problem-solving methods incorporated are still useful to us today.

Some instructors are brave enough to take advantage of a shared-governance idea in teaching their students. Students offer their input regarding the teaching (classroom/testing vs. seminar/term paper, etc.), methods of evaluation and, finally, a critique at the end of the term as to the effectiveness of the overall concept. Such a technique teaches students to take responsibility for themselves as well as allowing them to think creatively and independently. This does not mean replacing OB/GYN nursing with the Zen of Frisbee Throwing! It's a given that there are mandatory courses. However, the option lies with the means of conveying the subject matter to the pupil in the manner that will be most beneficial to the pupil.

Like all protégés, nursing students need role models. This is perhaps the most critical responsibility of the nurse educator. As health care reform becomes a reality, nurses will take on new commitments that will compel us to work with more self-reliance than in the past. In some instances, nurses will be the only medical advocates patients have.

Nursing educator Kathryn Vigen went public with an article that was published in the *Chicago Tribune* and the *Des Moines Register.* Vigen spoke for many when she said "Nurses prize true efficiency in caregiving, but have grown weary of administrators who say 'more efficient' when they mean 'more profitable'." Presently on leave from her position as head of nursing at Luther College, Vigen is directing a new graduate program for working nurses at Graceland College in Kansas City, Missouri. She realizes the power and strength of individuals working together for a common goal and urges her students to write letters, thereby recognizing their own worth and the value of their observations and opinions.

A mentor who sets an example with a strong, forthright, ethical attitude, who teaches the value of the self and who demonstrates caring through holistic nursing and empowerment is invaluable. This is particularly important today since the caliber of nursing student has changed significantly.

The Students

With the advent of two-year nursing programs, the type of student began to change from those attending three-year nursing schools. Those in the former lived at home, some were men, some were long out of high school, some were married with families. Those in three-year nursing schools were single women in their late teens, who were enjoying the last vestiges of youthful, carefree innocence and who boarded in dormitories at the school.

As the educational standards for nursing have shifted to encourage, if not demand, an undergraduate degree in the discipline, so, too, has the type of nursing student changed. As undergraduate degrees become a requirement for employment, three-year nursing schools have become dinosaurs, receding into a netherworld, a medical Jurassic Park. Those enrolling in college or university nursing programs today more closely resemble their colleagues from two-year programs. There is tremendous diversity in age. More men are applying and being accepted. Many of the women are married with families. For many, nursing is a second career. What we have, then, is a different breed of cat.

Although they still may be in awe of nursing and what nurses do, most students are not numbed by adolescent innocence. Students are sophisticated and not easily intimidated. These folks are not going to be lured into the "dumb-dumb" game where the nurse acts dumb so that the doctor will feel smart. Students have a sense of who and what they are about and they are not likely to tolerate absurdities that were once considered the norm. Many have well-defined ideas about the paths they wish to take in this profession. What is more important, many see nursing as a career rather than a job. This is especially true with the opportunities presented for nurses as physician assistants, nurse practitioners, legal consultants, sales or PR representatives for medical supply companies, home health care and research assistants.

Today's student is not satisfied with the basics that were acceptable years ago. Basics are good, but there is more to nursing now. New technologies demand more from nurses. There are more monitors, screens, and gauges. Many times I could see the advantage of a degree from MIT and the experience of moving heavy equipment for Bekins just to get a neurosurgery case started. Field work for PG&E would have been helpful also!

Extensive and varied education leaves nurses on a more equal footing with physicians. We have no problem addressing problems with physicians or taking the initiative and making decisions on our own.

Nursing students recognize and willingly take on the challenges they face. They must. If they don't, they won't survive. Nursing is an increasingly demanding profession that will not suffer the spineless gladly.

The nursing educational process requires cooperative respect among the primary players: the students, the educators, and the curriculum masters. The success of each is dependent on the other. More importantly, the success of the profession is contingent upon all three players. The changing face of health care demands not only that nurses are well educated and confident, but also that we possess the background and knowledge to explore the possibilities that exist for us outside the traditional role of hospital nurse.

CHAPTER TEN

What Are Our Options?

The Rose Garden: Many Thorns, Many Flowers

An experiment at Carondelet St. Mary's Hospital and Health Center in Tucson, Arizona allowed nurses to take on a managed care project and run it themselves. Phyllis Ethridge described the project in her article "Nurse-Run Managed Care?" (*American Journal of Nursing*, October 1990, p. 25). In the pre-managed care era of the 1980s, the hospital "...developed programs to empower the nursing staff, promote accountability and improve job satisfaction." The managed care aspect of the plan called for the establishment of "a professional nursing network with nurse case managers at the hub." Patients were referred to these case managers by varied sources ranging from nurses working in the hospital to physicians. Nurses were the primary care providers for patients, arranging for whatever treatment was needed. When services couldn't be provided through the network, payment was authorized to the appropriate provider. The ability to have immediate access to patients and initiate proper treatment and care "before their needs intensified… really chopped cost off at the front end."

A telephone interview in July 1994 with Phyllis Ethridge provided an update on this CNO (Community Nursing Organization). The average membership had grown to 15,000, at a cost of $3.85 per member per month. It was discovered that only 3% of Medicare recipients were receiving home care under the Medicare guidelines, whereas 6% needed home care.

The project was successful in "keeping patients from being admitted and re-admitted to the hospital." Patients were educated to identify early signs of problems. The result was a very low number of patient days, "almost 100% less than the number of days approved by the Health Care Financing Administration," noted Ethridge triumphantly. "Our goal," she added, "was to get in and get out."

As a result, Carondelet St. Mary's soon had four different contracts. In January 1994, it began a demonstration project that was awarded to them by HCFA. The most pleasing irony here is that, in this arena, Ethridge's CNO is competing with HMOs.

Many nurses are at a point in their professional lives where striking out in a new direction is not an option. As traditional nursing job opportunities diminish, the tentativeness of a once-secure career is disconcerting and frightening. For these individuals the glass is half empty. "Restructuring" cuts across all lines. Nurses who have been in their jobs for ten or twenty years are swept away as jobs are "redesigned" or they are compelled to apply again for their jobs that have been "redesigned." There is no guarantee that years of dedicated service will prevent the axe from falling. These nurses keep their fingers and toes crossed and hope they can dodge that axe until they are eligible to retire with benefits.

In some instances, nurses who are not ready for retirement, but who want to continue giving patient care, may consider working in an outpatient setting. Since the future in medicine seems to advocate the revolving door modus operandi, nurses may find this change less radical. For those accustomed to floor nursing, branching out to home health care might also be an alternative.

Those nurses who remain and survive the staff hacking are going to be in a brand new world. Their jobs will take on a supervisor's role (with little or no pay increase, to be sure!) that will involve responsibility for the actions of LVNs and CNAs. There will be very little interaction with patients except for a brief encounter, which might allow the RN a superficial assessment of those for whom he or she is ultimately responsible.

Nurses, individually and through their organizations, have issued a professional primal scream at this treacherous compromising of patient care. While deep down we might not mind handing over the scullery duties of the job (emptying bedpans, making beds, etc.), nurses also realize that it is during these chores we get to know our patients. It is through such ongoing contact that nurses pick up subtle changes, emotional and physical, that might hinder a patient's recovery. Matter-of-fact observations cannot be taken for granted. It's tough to rely on someone else to convey vital clues about a patient's condition. Such information requires education as well as experience. Consider the following:

> A care technician (is that generic enough?!) comes to the nursing station and says to the

nurse in charge, "Mrs. Redesign doesn't look too well."

"What seems to be the problem?"

"She's got a funny color and she's been sleeping for a long time."

"How was she when you bathed her?"

"She was sleeping all through her bath."

"Didn't you try to wake her?"

"Oh, no. I knew she had a bad night and that she needed her rest."

The nurse goes into Mrs. Redesign's room and sees that the patient has stopped breathing and that her face is turning a fashionable shade of blue. All of a sudden, it's time to put that ACLS (Advanced Cardiac Life Support) training into practice.

This might be excessively dramatic, but when the perspective is that the glass is half empty, it's necessary to pull out all the stops. As patient care is detrimentally altered, patients have less and less contact with their strongest advocates: the Registered Nurse.

Yet nursing, like many other professions, goes in cycles. Remember team nursing in the '60s? The new "redesign" concept is similar in structure, but not in quality of care due to the lack of registered nurses on the team. It might take several disasters similar the incident cited above to bring RNs back in the numbers that will ensure that patients get the kind of care they need.

Because of the modifications in the medical landscape, nurses who are looking ahead and wondering about careers may see ample and varied opportunities. The glass is half full for those who regard the various non-traditional avenues coming to the fore. Indeed, there are nurses who see nursing "as the best it's ever been. Our success story is unbelievable," Ingeborg Mauksch stated in her article "Will Nurses Contract Their Services?" (*American Journal of Nursing*, October 1990, p. 39). "We are finally valuing practice, valuing competence, and valuing the need to practice from a knowledge base," Mauksch continued. While these observations were noted four years ago, prior to the dramatic changes in health care, they are still quite valid today. Despite the negatives presented earlier in this book, nursing has made some dramatic strides as a profession.

Evidence of the progress the profession is making can be seen in several avenues. One of these is nurse intrapreneurship. Yes, **intra**preneurship. This option allows nurses to be creative and innovative within the institution of their employment. It is the intrapreneur who turns an idea into a money-making reality. This kind of enterprise is undertaken with (and at times, partially or totally underwritten by) the facility. Examples might include a psychiatric nurse who offers emergency counseling to individuals through a hospital emergency room, an operating room nurse who provides pre- and post-op consultations for patients and their families, a pediatric nurse involved with long term care who educates parents in caring for their child.

Nurses possess certain qualities that make intrapreneurship a natural course. We have solid all-around knowledge of patient care. Our daily dealings with the patient allow us to assess unmet needs or areas where improvement is necessary. Our patients' needs come before our own, thereby engendering an atmosphere of trust. Yet, this is no guarantee for success. Intrapreneurs must possess some significant attributes if they are to succeed. Any new idea, no matter how terrific, requires research and perseverance. All parties and/or departments that might be involved should be consulted. Assertiveness, time-management skills, flexibility, political astuteness, patience, and a true passion for the innovative are all critical to its success. A well-thought-out plan carefully presented will go much further than one brought up during conversation as "Oh, by the way, I was just thinking..."

Nurse intrapreneurs realize great personal satisfaction and increased financial compensation. Their fiscal risk is shared with the facility, which has an established reputation. The nurse also has the benefit of being in an institution that has a strong employee/referral base as well as access to the many programs a medical center or hospital offers.

The organization also benefits by encouraging the creativity of its employees. Such innovations might make the facility more accessible to many more people and the word of mouth "Did you know the Can Do No Wrong Medical Center is now offering consulting services for all new parents? for parents with children who need special orthopedic care? for chocoholics? (sponsored by Godiva chocolates!!)" In her article, "Nurse Intrapreneurs: The Heroes of Health Care's Future" (*Nursing Outlook*, January/February 1991), author Jo Manion noted that "nurses. . .are the health professionals who routinely serve as the key link for the entire health care team. This positions nurses for significant intrapreneurial opportunities."

The Resumé: Information Highway to a New Career

In the past it was enough for a nurse to show up at an interview in a crisp clean uniform and newly polished shoes. It wasn't a matter of whether the job was available, it was more on the order of can you start this minute (yesterday would have been even better!). Well, there's good news and bad news. The good news is that the uniform and shoes are out; the bad news is that the resumé is in—big time.

A resumé is a synopsis of your life and your achievements. It lists your education and work experience and provides employers a glimpse of your community activities and recreational interests. It also allows employers to see what organizations, professional or otherwise, in which you have membership. This, together with a dynamite cover letter and a dazzling interview will get your foot and your entire body in the door.

It is critical that information on the resumé be geared for the job to which you are applying. If you have experience in flower arranging and manure shoveling and you're applying for a job on a ranch, all the manure information needs to be up front where the rancher can see it first. Flower arranging goes to the bottom where it will be seen as an aside. Someone with journalism experience and medical insurance expertise who is interested in a position in an insurance company editing their weekly newsletter would put the journalism information first, with the insurance background second. All of this background is important and pertinent to the job under consideration.

Professional organizations that are relevant to the job should also be at the forefront under that specific heading, as should community service and volunteer experience. For example, someone looking at a managerial position would want to highlight any volunteer service that involved chairing a fund-raiser or big charity event. Such experience speaks to leadership and organizing capabilities.

At a seminar I recently attended, the speaker who discussed resumés commented that "the more initials you have after your name, the better. This refers to titles, certifications, educational degrees, etc.—RN, ACLS, CNOR, BSN, MSN, PhD, JD, AMEN. You get the picture!

Resumés are not as formidable as they might seem. If you're putting one together for the first time, it can be quite an ego booster. When all your achievements are laid out on paper in an organized way, it's nice to step back: "Hm, not bad. I didn't realize I'd done all this!"

Libraries and bookstores offer a wide selection of books on how to go about formulating a resumé. Also, there are counselors and consultants who can assist you in completing this condensed version of your life.

Remember: Your resumé is an employer's first introduction to you so it has to be fabulous. (OK, OK, well done will suffice!)

The New Age of Nursing: Variations on a Theme

Nurse practitioners and physician assistants have played prominent roles in medicine in the last decade. In rural areas particularly, there is a push for nurse practitioners to assume more responsibilities such as writing prescriptions for medications and admitting patients to hospitals. Not surprisingly, this has evoked a great deal of wailing and whining from the physician sector, which perceives this extension of duties as an infringement on its closely guarded domain. Indeed, open war has been declared between the American Medical Association (representing the hallowed halls of medicine) and the American Nurses Association (fighting for the autonomy and progression of nurse practitioners).

As nurse practitioners seek more autonomy and responsibility to insure the wellness of the patients in their care, they are also fighting for direct reimbursement from insurance companies, Medicare, and Medicaid for the services they render. If the idea of nurses writing prescriptions has physicians upset, the prospect of nurses receiving direct reimbursement has them hysterical. Doctors see their long-standing empire crumbling and they feel a sense of helplessness as they fight over issues that are compelling them to relinquish coveted control.

Working as a physician assistant (PA) allows for a different sort of independence than working as a nurse practitioner. Under the direct supervision of specific physicians, PAs usually take medical histories, conduct physical examinations, order lab tests, change dressings, perform minor procedures, counsel and educate patients on health matters. Like the nurse practitioner, the focus of the physician assistant is wellness.

To work as either an NP or a PA requires additional college study or enrollment in a specialized program. Local medical centers or colleges/universities can provide appropriate information.

Insurance companies, Health Maintenance Organizations (HMO), and Preferred Provider Organizations (PPO) hire nurses in any of the following areas: Pre-Admission Review,

Discharge Planning, Peer Review, Utilization Review, Case Management, and Quality Assurance. Whereas classifieds for Med-Surg or OB or CCU nurses have declined, there are increasing numbers of insurance company ads for nurses sprouting up in the paper. Not only insurance companies, but also hospitals are calling for nurses to fill these positions. Nursing journals and magazines are excellent sources of information for continuing education courses and "how to" seminars in such specialties. For additional information, write or call:

National Association of Health Care Quality
5700 Old Orchard Road
First Floor
Skokie, IL 60077
(708) 966-9392

As baby boomers get older and more feeble, there will be ample employment in long-term care. For those baby boomers who refuse to acknowledge the limitations of age and insist upon enjoying the antics of youth—in-line skating, skateboarding, motorcycle riding, walking, etc., rehabilitation services will prove invaluable! Rehabilitation nursing will be a thriving specialty assisting those approaching the Centrum Silver years with reckless abandon. Master's degrees in rehabilitative nursing are offered in six universities throughout the United States: the University of Alabama at Birmingham, Rush University in Chicago, Thomas Jefferson University in Philadelphia, the State of New York University at Buffalo, Columbia University in New York and the University of Texas in Arlington.

For further information on rehabilitation nursing, contact:

American Congress of Rehabilitation Medicine
5700 Old Orchard Road, First Floor
Skokie, IL 60077-1057
(708) 966-3433

Association of Rehabilitation Nurses
5700 Old Orchard Road, First Floor
Skokie, IL 60077-1057
(708) 966-3433

Medical Rehabilitation Education Foundation
1910 Association Drive, Suite 200
Reston, VA 22091
(703) 648-9350 or (800) 368-3513

Energetic nurses with some business savvy might want to take a look at what the business world has to offer. Medical and pharmaceutical companies frequently seek nurses for sales and marketing positions. Such pursuits allow companies to tap into the medical expertise and experience nurses possess. For their part, nurses realize a tremendous amount of autonomy in such roles. Marketing, which frequently crosses over into public relations, tests creative talents that previous jobs might not have entertained. Nurses investigating these areas might find networking especially helpful. Contact:

National Nurses in Business Association (NNBA)
1000 Burnett Avenue, Suite 450
Concord, CA 94520
(510) 356-2642

For information about marketing, contact:

Academy for Health Services Marketing (AHSM)
c/o American Marketing Association
250 S. Wacker Drive, Suite 200
Chicago, IL 60606
(312) 648-0536

American Society for Health Care Marketing
& Public Relations (ASHCMPR)
American Hospital Association
840 N. Lake Shore Drive
Chicago, IL 60611
(800) 621-6712

Medical-legal nurse consulting is a growing field. Since it was founded in 1989 by 35 RNs, the Association of Legal Nurse Consultants (AALNC) membership had grown to 700 nurses by 1992. One does not need to be a lawyer or have a legal background to pursue this career change. A nursing background alone suffices to consider one an expert on nursing standards of care. Workshops and seminars are available to prepare nurses to enter this specialized field. For information, contact:

American Association of Legal Nurse
Consultants
500 North Michigan Avenue, Suite 1400
Chicago, IL 60611-3796
(312) 670-0550

Carondelet Management Institute
2090 N. Kolb Road, #100
Tucson, AZ 85715-4055
(800) 726-3888

In the area of biotechnology, nurses are hired to assist "...in research, compiling and verifying data, and assisting with trials of the product. Some companies like to send nurses out to demonstrate a new product to physicians or other health care members... to insure its proper use" (Estela, Linda *Alternative Careers in Nursing*, Hayward, CA: Nurses Research Publications, 1993). Jobs in biotechnology may be stressful because workers have to deal with the unhappy consumer. Tact and diplomatic skills are definitely necessary!

Medical writing is also an alternative, especially if one is content to work in the quiet of one's home. There are opportunities in local newspapers, radio, and television stations. If one craves the stimulation of camaraderie while at work, writing for high-tech, educational, or pharmaceutical companies might be worth exploring. Nurses can acquire information from the following sources:

American Medical Writers Association
(AMWA)
9650 Rockville Pike
Bethesda, MD 20814

The Society for Technical Communication
815 Fifteenth Street, N.W., Suite 506
Washington, DC 20005

Health Sciences Communications Association
(HESCA)
6105 Lindell Boulevard
St. Louis, MO 63112
(314) 725-4722

Additional references regarding the "how to's" of writing are provided in Appendix B.

For individuals who are free of confining responsibilities—husbands, children, mortgages, goldfish, etc.—working outside the United States may have tremendous appeal. Employment opportunities are available through international business, the World Health Organization, the Peace Corps and Project Hope. Of course, the military offers travel as well as the chance to be "all that you can be."

Saudi Arabia recruits health care workers through the following:

Kama Enterprise, Inc.
4380 Southwest Macadam Avenue, Suite 490
Portland, OR 97201
(800) 433-7791 (*Careers,* p. 69)

Those who wish to become involved in culturally diverse nursing, such as working with a specific ethnic population (Asian Americans, North American Indians, Russian immigrants, etc.), may refer to Appendix C for a listing of contacts.

Cement Mixer Philosophy

Years ago Kaiser cement trucks were pastel pink and had the slogan "Find a need and fill it!" emblazoned on the side.

Close to 20,000 nurses in the United States have adopted this philosophy and turned their medical knowledge into thriving businesses. These are the nursing entrepreneurs. Often stultified professionally and stagnating financially, these folks have taken a deep breath and moved into areas that will provide more prestige and larger incomes. They want to be out of the hospital, out of the clinic, and on their own.

These are people who are tired of depending on others for recognition and tired of waiting for administration and physicians to get with the program and give them more autonomy, more responsibility and fewer excuses. These individuals have looked around, recognized problems and mentally calculated solutions. They are ready to be on their own and put their ideas into action. The main advantage here is that these nurses are staying within a familiar world. It does take courage to go off and fulfill a dream, but remaining within a known discipline can somewhat cushion the blow. At least one is not starting at ground zero.

For some, nursing isn't all it's cracked up to be, and the sooner it's left behind, the better. Career fantasies lurk in the back of our minds. How often have we thought about and longed for the occasion or excuse to present itself so that we might break free from nursing and put into action the secret dreams we've harbored for so long.

Is It Time to Buy a Flower Shop?

The American poet Carl Sandburg noted, "Nothing happens unless first a dream." When it comes to changing careers or making a dream a reality, a great deal of courage and planning are required. Unlike many jobs, dreams involve something we *like* to do. Perhaps it revolves around a hobby or a special interest: flower arranging, photography, crafts, etc. Radical career changes can be made without financial investment. If peace of mind overrides financial considerations, several options are available. One can offer photography skills to a newspaper, a business or a magazine. Caffeine fiends may find their calling at a local cafe and chocoholics might find great satisfaction working behind the counter of a neighborhood candy store. At the other end of the calorie spectrum, an individual who has successfully completed a diet program may find great satisfaction in working for a similar organization as a counselor.

Some career changes may require additional education. Most often this can be achieved through evening classes, thereby allowing one to remain in a current position without compromising income. Master's programs offer the necessary education to advance or branch out within the current profession or move on to a new direction. Often, the dream held dear is one of complete self-sufficiency. It is the dream of entrepreneurship.

> Nothing was ever achieved without enthusiasm.
>
> —*Ralph Waldo Emerson*

The dream may be the spark to get things going, but there are specific characteristics that are essential to make a good entrepreneur. Before you get caught up in the dream, take a good look at yourself and ask the following questions:

- ➢ Are you willing to take moderate risks?
- ➢ Do you have enough money in the bank to carry you for several months?
- ➢ Do you have mental and physical resiliency?
- ➢ Do you possess determination and perseverance?
- ➢ Do you have interpersonal skills that will allow you to work with the public?
- ➢ Do you need to control and direct?
- ➢ Do you have a need for achievement? (Vogel, 1988)

Besides the information the above self-examination will elicit, it is also necessary to take an inventory of business and management skills and personal characteristics. An honest assessment of these areas should help determine whether you are suited to an entrepreneurial undertaking. You will then have a better idea whether you should open that flower shop you've been dreaming about or move to Pittsburgh and become a welder!

It Takes Money, Honey

Any dream remains a dream without the proper finances to back it up. This means not only the money to start up the business, but also some serious bucks to keep it afloat until you get established. It's hard to paint a picture of success when poor planning has left you poverty-stricken. As a friend of mine once said: "Being poor is romantic for about two weeks!"

The idea then, is to have enough money in the bank to carry you through the early period. Those starting out in real estate are advised to have enough savings available to support themselves for six months to a year. This is a good point of departure. It allows you to concentrate on your new enterprise without worrying about money.

Frugality should be the rule at this time (the things you can do with Hamburger Helper!), but there will also be occasions when it will be necessary to take a potential client or customer out to lunch or dinner. In such instances, it's appropriate to go to a very good restaurant, not necessarily the most expensive restaurant in town.

Startup costs for a new business can be prohibitive, especially for some franchises. Don't let the dream carry you away. Be realistic. Don't get yourself into hock by mortgaging your home, your dog, and your firstborn.

Do your research. There are plenty of books in the library and at the bookstore on the subject of starting a new business, a small business. Talk to those who are already on their own. Talk to the potential competition. See what organizations can offer assistance. Touch bases with the local chamber of commerce. Attend lunches held by small business associations, and start doing some networking. The pieces of the puzzle are there, it's up to you to sort through them and put the picture together.

Realizing a dream requires that you have your eyes open. This will allow you to comprehend the situation realistically and minimize the possibilities of disappointment and failure.

CHAPTER ELEVEN

The Starting Point: Me

Playing With Pronouns: The I's Have It!

Within each of us is that facet of human nature that cries, "Me! Me! Me!" Sigmund Freud called it ego. Your mother (and my mother!) calls it selfish and self-centered. The word moguls of the 90s label it self-absorbed, and your friends (not to mention your enemies) refer to this very core of your being as boring. All of these tags are valid, and with the exception of Freud's ego, all are subjective and negative. Individuals in today's society spew out sentences littered with the words I, me, and mine. It is one of life's great joys to talk about oneself. Such talk confirms identity and bolsters self-worth.

> We helpers deserve to nurture ourselves as well as those we care for. Some caregivers think that to sacrifice and suffer is spiritual. I believe this might be called "spiritual anorexia."
>
> —*Caryn Summers, RN*

For nurses, the attainment of self-worth is the first stop of a journey that can eventually unify the profession. Ironically, through the "Me! Me! Me!" syndrome, nurses can come to grips with the fabulous and caring people that we are. As we come to recognize how invaluable we really are, we will understand our value to the group—our profession—as a whole.

Our maturation as individuals is a process that may begin with any of the following:

- "I am wonderful!"
- "I am terrific!"
- "Did you see what I did?"
- "I saved that patient's life through my quick thinking and expertise."
- "I am somebody."

Yet, by our very nature, nurses turn outward. As we evolve, we will look around and ask:

- "What can I do to help?"
- "What can I do for you?"
- "How can I get involved?"

Nurses who are confident look beyond the self. We become aware, we educate ourselves, and most of all, we become involved.

The Big Groan: Political Awareness and/or Involvement

It is crucial that during these turbulent (albeit exciting) times, we maintain an acute comprehension of all that is going on around us. Legislation is presented on an ongoing basis that is bound to have a profound effect on the ways we practice our craft—direct reimbursement of nursing services rendered, scope of practice laws, etc.

Perhaps the most painless way to be politically aware is to join and become active in any of a number of appropriate nursing organizations. On a national level, there is the American Nurses Association and the National League of Nursing. Each state has its own organization, which serves its immediate membership. In addition, most specialties have organizations, e.g., AORN (Association of Operating Room Nurses).

These associations and organizations work at the national and state levels to lobby for or against the bills that will affect us. Most importantly, they provide journals and newsletters, usually on a monthly basis, which reveal political insights and furnish valuable articles on the state of nursing today.

In addition, there are numerous other nursing journals and magazines, some of which are specialized (*Nurse Management, Nursing Education*). Others are more general—*Nursing Outlook, Revolution: The Journal of Nurse Empowerment*— and offer information on current nursing concerns.

On a more personal level, a political novice may want to start out in familiar territory: the hospital. You might be able serve on quality assurance and joint practice committees, personnel and restructuring committees. Nurses might also seek out seats on hospital boards.

Also, you can become involved politically at the local level and make your voice heard in that arena. Those who are more aggressive might want to enter politics at the state level or become a lobbyist on behalf of your local nursing organization.

Especially effective in an election year is starting up or participating in letter-writing campaigns to legislators on behalf of whatever act or bill is on the floor and requires specific numbers of votes to pass or fail (depending on your viewpoint).

Nevertheless, politics is more than the cliché of hefty bureaucrats puffing on big cigars in dimly lit restaurants, negotiating the future of the population as they pound back their three martinis. Being political means having opinions and expressing them. This can be approached in several ways and requires nothing more than observation.

Several years ago, one of the networks put on a series, a sitcom, about nurses: *Nightingales.* It was stereotypical and insulting, depicting nurses as muddleheaded bimbos in provocative uniforms. Nurses' organizations waged a campaign to let the network executives know that their program was unacceptable gibberish. Nurses also assaulted the media, effecting a tremendous letter writing campaign that clogged mailrooms throughout the country. Ultimately, the show was canceled. The campaign was apparently effective, but the show was also so terrible it probably would have been canceled anyway. Nevertheless, nurses took a stand, loud and clear. There was no misunderstanding.

Earlier in this book, I mentioned the work *Grievous Sin* by mystery writer Faye Kellerman. The author's characterizations of nurses left me irate enough to write her explaining my displeasure. Subsequently, I received a response from Ms. Kellerman. She carefully assured me that she held nurses in very high regard. However, as a mystery writer, it was necessary for her to create individuals with distasteful personae to make the story believable.

Our correspondence achieved two things: I let the author know that many of her fans might be nurses who are very aware of and sensitive to negative portrayals. Ms. Kellerman provided me with a novelist's perspective that I will consider the next time I read a similar book. This reciprocal educational process is an example of what can be achieved on an individual basis.

The news can also be a source of misunderstanding and misinformation. Is the reporting of a nurses' strike accurate? If not, call the station and tell them to be more evenhanded. Is a series in the local newspaper appropriate? Is it fair to nurses? Does it use nurses as valid sources of knowledge. Would you like to see a medical column by a nurse in the daily paper? Let the editors know. Letters to the editor are another means of drawing the public's attention to an article of questionable taste. If something upsets you, send a letter to the editor. If nothing else, it's a good way to vent your anger and frustration!

Some newspapers have special slots set aside in their editorial section for freelance pieces. This is a great vehicle to let people know what is going on in medicine, in the hospital, and in nursing. Such pieces do not need to be lengthy, just direct and to the point.

Finally, there is *the mouth*! We all have one and we all know how to use it! If you are a member of a book club, an investment club, a knitting club, you can get your message across in everyday conversation. It's not necessary to hit your friends over the head with a two-by-four, but you can bring them up-to-date with a few well-chosen comments. Encourage their opinions. Make them aware.

CHAPTER TWELVE

Pulling It All Together

The Transition: From I to We, From Me to Us

There are more than 2 million nurses in the United States. That's all of us--men, women, gays, straights, tall, short, chunky, thin, blondes, brunettes, redheads, balds. Think about it. That's a lot of clout and a good number of votes. If we worked together as a single unit for the betterment of our profession, we would be unstoppable.

Need, anger, and frustration are proving to be compelling catalysts to unite nurses. In 1985, faced with having no representation for their collective bargaining unit, nurses at Lenox Hill Hospital in New York City pulled together and established their own independent nurses union. This effort was achieved by making the staff aware of the leadership's strength and their plans for the future. This victory required tenacity and cooperation as the newly founded union defeated the older, established District 1199 of the Retail, Wholesale Department

Store Union (which had previously represented the nurses), and the New York State Nurses Association. Once elections were held and disputes were settled by the NLRB, the nurses' union met with hospital officials and negotiated a contract that offered a great deal to the nurses.

Our power as a unit was never more evident than on March 31, 1995, when close to 25,000 nurses marched as a group in Washington, DC, to bring the hazards of nursing layoffs to the nation's attention. The march was initiated by the publishers of *Revolution—The Journal of Nurse Empowerment.* However, as Joni Ketter observed, it didn't take long for the American Nurses Association "to protest the replacement of registered nurses at the bedside by unlicensed and minimally trained personnel as hospitals restructure to reduce costs and increase profits" (*The American Nurse,* April/May 1995). Many nurses who had been refused the time off to attend the rally jeopardized their job security by attending anyway.

Despite the rallying cry for unity, nurses still tend to remain fragmented, each of us concerned about our own niche and our particular specialty. It's time to come together as the powerful entity that we are. Let's get on with the business of caring for our patients. Let's stand up to protect ourselves. There is no better time than now.

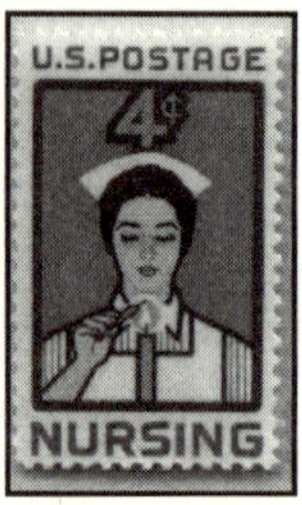

U.S. Postage stamp, released in the 1960s, depicts a positive, although idealized, image of nurses.

Tomorrow: Weaving the Dream

Writer and philosopher Henry David Thoreau said "If one advances confidently in the direction of his dreams, and endeavors to live the life which he has imagined, he will meet with a success unexpected in common hours."

Indeed, to dream is to hope for and seek a better reality. Martin Luther King dreamed of racial equality. Aristotle Onasis dreamed of financial success. Anne Frank dreamed of freedom.

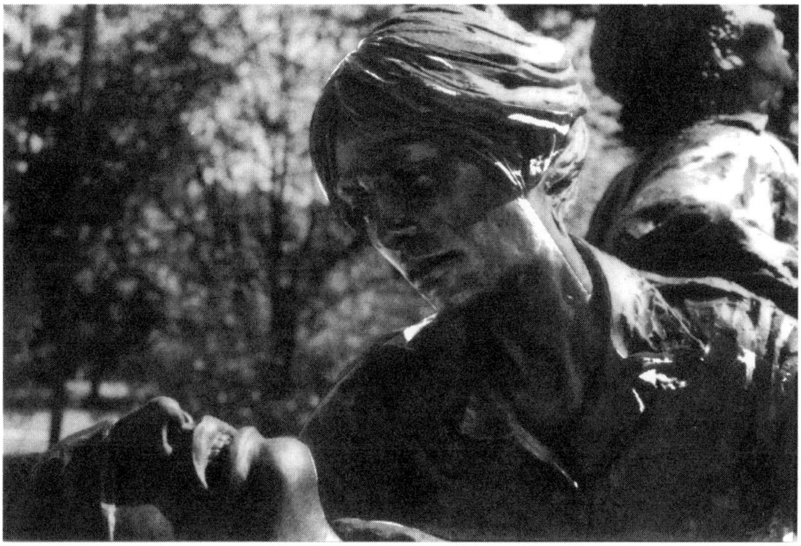

The Vietnam Women's Memorial in Washington, DC, is a tribute to the women who served in that war, many of whom were nurses. Their faces show their pain, compassion and integrity.

Nurses can dream also: that we can rise above our prescribed image and think well of ourselves, that we can pull together as a cohesive profession.

The changes in health care in this country may be the very catalyst that transforms many of our dreams into realities. Consider the following: a hospital owned and operated by the nurses who work there, where patients are the priority and abusive doctors are not tolerated, where everyone works together for the welfare of the patients and whose efforts are rewarded through profit-sharing. This is a dream to be sure, but it's a very pleasant departure from the reality of today's medicine. While we may not own the hospitals in which we work (yet!), we still can tell our patients:

"We're here for you. We're on your side just as we've always been. There may not be as many of us in the hospitals any more, but now we're going where we can do the most good. We're coming to you in the community, to make sure you *stay* well. As always, when you need us, we'll be there."

APPENDIX A

Nursing's Agenda For Health Care Reform

Nursing's plan for reform converts a system that focuses on the costly treatment of illness to a system that emphasizes primary health care services and the promotion, restoration and maintenance of health. It sets forth new delivery arrangements that make health care a more vital part of individual and community life.

A Health Care System in Crisis

More than two million nurses in America are at the front lines. What nurses see are the alarming effects of a system that has lost touch with the communities it's supposed to serve.

Today, more than 60 million Americans are either uninsured or underinsured. Now the system's inability to contain costs is placing more and more Americans with "adequate" insurance coverage at risk of hardship when major illnesses do occur.

If the system remains unchanged, spending will reach between \$2.1 and \$2.7 trillion by the year 2000 (National Leadership Coalition for Health Care Reform, 1991, "A Comprehensive Reform Plan for the Health Care System," p. 2).

The Framework for Change

Nurses strongly believe that the health care system must be restructured, reoriented, and decentralized to guarantee access to services, contain costs, and ensure quality care. Our plan provides central control in the form of federal minimum standards for essential services and federally defined eligibility requirements.

The cornerstone for nursing's plan for reform is the delivery of primary health care services to households and individuals in convenient, familiar places.

Consumers must be the focus of the health care system. Individuals must be given incentives to assume more responsibility for their health. Promotion of healthy lifestyles and better informed consumer decisions can contribute to effective and economical health care delivery.

In implementing reforms, attention must be directed to the unique needs of special population groups whose health care needs have been neglected (e.g., AIDS victims and those who have difficulty securing insurance because of pre-existing conditions).

Coverage of pregnant women and children is critical. The first step represents a cost effective investment in the future health and prosperity of the nation.

It is this set of values that distinguishes nursing's plan from other proposals and offers a realistic approach to health care reform.

A Plan for Reform

Nursing's plan for health care reform shifts the emphasis of the health care system from illness and cure to wellness and care. It sets forth new strategies for guaranteeing universal coverage; making health care a more vital part of community life; and ensuring that the health care services provided are appropriate, effective, and cost efficient.

It envisions a standard package of essential health care services and the manner in which these services are delivered. By taking this approach, traditional illness services are balanced with provisions for health maintenance services prevent illness, reduce cost, and avoid institutionalization.

The ultimate goal will be, over time, to merge all government-sponsored health programs into a single public program.

Coverage Options

Universal coverage for the federally defined package of essential services will be provided through an integration of public and private plans and resources.

- A public plan, administered by the states, will provide coverage for the poor (those below 200% of the federal poverty level), high-risk populations, and the potentially medically indigent. Any employer or individual will also have the option of buying into this plan as their source of coverage.

- Private plans will be required to offer, at a minimum, the nationally standardized package of essential services.

All citizens and residents will be required to be covered by one of these options. No one will be denied insurance because of pre-existing conditions. If employers do not offer private coverage, they will be required to pay into thc public plan for their employees.

Premiums and Payment Rates

Access to health care services will be enhanced by offering insurance premiums that the public can afford and payment rates to providers that are equitable and inclusive.

Because providers will be reimbursed fairly through insurance and the problems of uncompensated care will be largely eliminated, there will be no need for providers to charge consumers amounts above the established rate.

Special programs will provide services and outreach to vulnerable populations to compensate for formerly inadequate care and its consequences.

Nursing's plan seeks to prevent impoverishment and the potential loss of dignity by recognizing both public responsibility for long-term care and continued personal commitment to planning for such care. Financing arrangements will provide "front-end" coverage for chronic care and long-term care services of short duration through a variety of public and private options.

Length and/or intensity of illness may generate catastrophic costs. Limits will be placed on individuals' out-of-pocket payments for catastrophic health care expenses. Costs to insurers or individuals that exceed preset limits will be covered through a state reinsurance pool, to which all insurers must contribute.

Delivery mechanisms for health services will be decentralized in terms of planning and administration to foster greater consumer orientation. States will have the authority to modify implementation to reflect geographical diversity.

The wider use of a range of qualified health professionals will increase access to care, particularly in understaffed specialties, such as primary health care, and in underserved urban and rural geographical areas. It will also facilitate selection of the most cost-effective option for care.

Nursing's plan envisions managed care as organized delivery systems that link the financing of health care to the delivery of services.

Managed care must be restructured to retain the maximum possible consumer choice and to place a premium on services that address the health of consumers.

The aim of case management is to make health care less fragmented and more holistic for those individuals with complex health care needs. A variety of health care professionals are qualified to provide this service. The first allegiance of these providers will be to their clients. They will provide direct care and negotiate with systems on behalf of their clients.

A Realistic Plan of Action

Universal coverage will be achieved through implementation of both public and private plan options. Employers will be motivated to collaborate with employees in shaping private plans that best satisfy their needs. It may be necessary to expand coverage to segments of the population in sequential steps.

The first targeted population would include all pregnant women, children under age six, and those individuals who demonstrate a health status seriously compromised by a history of inadequate care. Other segments of the population would be covered as quickly as possible.

The process will culminate with the merge of all entitlement plans into a single public program to provide coverage to all citizens and residents who do not have or cannot obtain coverage through a private plan.

The Fiscal Implications of Reform

It is impossible to predict the dollar amount that will be associated with the expansion of services or the efficiencies in nursing's plan.

A number of proposals for reform have been introduced. Among those proposals with cost estimates, additional health care costs range from $60-$90 billion (*The Pepper Commission, A Call for Action: A Final Report,* September 1990, p. 137., Mark G. Battle, January 8, 1991, National Association of Social Workers, remarks during NASW's National Health Care Press Conference.). While nursing's plan for expanded coverage is similar to some of these proposals, offsetting proposed efficiencies integral to the plan will create significant dollars for reallocation.

Extension of coverage for essential services to the uninsured and underinsured will result in the dedication of more dollars. It will also be necessary to dedicate more dollars to the expansion of long-term care services. Nursing's plan, however, calls for more limited coverage supported through a combination of public dollars and enhanced personal responsibility.

In the initial phases of nursing's health care reform, the emphasis on preventive services will require dollars. Over time, however, improved health resulting from the availability of comprehensive primary health care services will produce a cost-reducing "health dividend."

Cost Savings

New costs associated with nursing's plan will be offset to a considerable degree by the following cost-saving initiatives:

- Required usage of managed care in the public plan and encouraged use in private plans.
- Controlled growth of the health care system through planning and prudent resource allocation.
- Assurance of direct access to a full range of qualified providers.
- Incentives for consumers and providers to be more cost efficient in selecting health care options.
- Elimination of unnecessary bureaucratic controls and administrative procedures, through such measures as standardized billing, simplified utilization review, streamlined administrative procedures, regulatory reforms, and consolidation of plans.

Sources of Revenue

Responsibility for financing health care reform must be distributed equitably among individuals, employers, and government.

Individuals will continue to pay a portion of health costs through copayments by households and individuals with incomes above 200% of the poverty level.

Employers will provide private health insurance that meets or exceeds minimum federal standards for their employees and dependents, or will provide coverage through the public plan. Accommodations will be made to provide small businesses with the necessary financial relief to meet this obligation.

Nursing's health care reform plan calls for consolidation of existing government health plans into a single public program.

A Look Toward The Future

To be most effective, a health care system must do more than provide equipment, supplies, facilities, and personnel. It must guarantee universal access to an assured standard of care. It must use health resources effectively and efficiently—balancing efforts to promote health with the capacity to cure disease. It must provide care in convenient, familiar locations. Also, it must make full use of the range of qualified health professionals and diverse settings for care. It is this insight that underlies nursing's plan for reform—making it the most viable solution to the nation's health care crisis.

This abridged version of *Nursing's Agenda for Health Care Reform* has been approved by the American Nurses Association for publication in this book.

The unabridged version of the *Agenda* may be obtained by contacting:

American Nurses Publishing
600 Maryland Avenue, SW
Suite 100 West
Washington, DC 20024-2571
Tel: (202) 554-4444

Note: 62 nursing organizations support *Nursing's Agenda for Health Care Reform*

APPENDIX B

Resources For Writers

American Heritage Dictionary of the English Language, 3rd edition. Boston: Houghton Mifflin, 1992.

American Psychological Association. *Publication Manual of the American Psychological Association,* 4th edition. Washington, DC, 1994.

The Associated Press Staff, *Associated Press Stylebook and Libel Manual: The Journalist's Bible,* Menlo Park. CA: Addison-Wesley, 1994.

Chapman, R. L. Ed. *Roget's International Thesaurus,* 5th edition. New York: Harper Collins, 1992.

Chicago Editorial Staff, *The Chicago Manual of Style,* 14th edition. Chicago: University of Chicago Press, 1993.

Dillard, A. *The Writing Life,* New York: Harper Collins, 1990.

Fondiller, S. H. & Nerone, B. J. *Health Professionals Stylebook: Putting Your Language to Work* (NLN Pub. No. 14—2551). New York: National League for Nursing, 1993.

Fondiller, S. H. *The Writer's Workbook* (NLN Pub. No. 14—2470). New York, National League for Nursing, 1992.

Gordon, K. E. *The Transitive Vampire*, New York: Times Books, 1984.

Johnson, E. D. *The Handbook of Good English*, New York: Washington Square Press, 1991.

Lewis, J. *The New York Times Manual of Style and Usage*, New York: Random House, 1982.

Raimes, A. *Grammar Troublespots: An Editorial Guide for Students*, New York: St. Martin's, 1992.

Strunk, W., Jr., and White, E. B. *The Elements of Style*, 3rd edition. New York: Macmillan, 1979.

Warriner, J. E., et al. *English Grammar and Composition*, Heritage edition. New York: Harcourt Brace Jovanovich, 1978.

APPENDIX C

Multi-Cultural Nursing

The following is a list of facilities that provide culturally diverse nursing opportunities.

Arthur G. James Cancer Hospital & Research Institute
Columbus OH
Kelly Pifer
(614) 293-3047

Beth Israel Health Care System
New York NY
Mae G. Concannon, RN
Assistant Director of Human Resources

Brackenridge Hospital —
Children's Hospital of Austin
Austin TX
Jane Fannin
Nurse Recruiter
1-800-880-0038

Fairfax Hospital
Falls Church VA
Nurse Recruitment
1-800-234-4405
(703) 698-3298 (Virginia)

Harborview Medical Center
Seattle WA
Nurse Recruitment
1-800-443-6793
(206) 223-5963

KAMA Enterprises, Inc.
Portland OR
Kim or Chris
Dept. AJN-7
1-800-247-8590

Mayo Medical Center
Rochester MN
Nurse Recruitment
1-800-247-8590

Miami Children's Hospital
Miami FL
Karen Nesbitt, RN
Nurse Recruiter
1-800-955-6511

Michael Reese Hospital &
Medical Center
Chicago IL
Paul Walden
(312) 791-3049

Mount Auburn Hospital
Cambridge MA
Maureen Donohue
Employment Services
(617) 499-5082

MultiCare Medical Center
Tacoma WA
24-hour Job Line:
(206) 552-1256

National Black Nurses' Association, Inc.
Washington DC
(202) 393-6870

National Institutes of Health Clinical Center
Bethesda MD
Nursing Department
1-800-732-5985

New England Sinai Hospital/Rehabilitation Center
Stoughton MA
Health Care Recruiter
(617) 297-1197/8

New York Foundling Hospital
New York NY
Nurse Recruiter

Our Lady of the Resurrection Medical Center
Chicago IL
Nurse Recruitment
(312) 282-7000 ext. 3708

Phoenix Memorial Hospital
Phoenix AZ
Human Resources
Call collect:
(602) 258-5111 ext. 283

Rockford Memorial Hospital
Rockford IL
Sue Potter
(815) 961-6110

St. Joseph Hospital
Denver CO
Personnel
1-800-345-5559

The Toledo Hospital
Toledo OH
Jill Kooyers
(419) 471-3746

Tri-City Medical Center
Oceanside CA
Human Resources
1-800-727-TCMC ext. 7130

UNC Hospitals
Chapel Hill NC
Patricia L. Jones, RN
or Kay Lytle

University Community Hospital
Tampa FL
Human Resources Dept.
1-800-998-6550

University Hospital of Cleveland
Cleveland OH
Sioban McGreal
(216) 844-1686

USC University Hospital
Los Angeles CA
Karen Blacklund
Human Resources Dept.
1-800-955-6515

WSKC Dialysis Services
Oak Park IL
Kathryn Kelly
(708) 386-2511 ext. 276

Yale New Haven Hospital
New Haven CT
Human Resources Dept.
Clinical Recruitment Division

APPENDIX D

International And National Health Organizations

Alpha Tau Delta National
Fraternity for
Professional Nurses
14631 N Second Drive
Phoenix AZ 85023

American Association for
Respiratory Therapy
1720 Regal Row
Dallas TX 75235

American Association of
Colleges of Nursing
1 Dupont Circle
Suite 530
Washington D.C. 20036

American Association of
Diabetes Educators
Box 56
N. Woodbury Rd.
Pittman NJ 08071

American Cancer Society
777 Third Avenue
New York NY 10017

American Diabetes
Association
600 Fifth Avenue
New York NY 10020

American Heart Association
840 North Lakeshore Drive
Chicago IL 60611

American Hospital
Association
840 North Lakeshore Drive
Chicago IL 60611

American Lung Association
1740 Broadway
New York NY 10019

American Medical Society
535 North Dearborn Street
Chicago IL 60610

American Nurses
Association
600 Maryland Avenue, SW
Suite 100W
Washington DC 20024

American Organization of
Nurse Executives
840 Lakeshore Drive
Chicago IL 60611

American Public Health
Association
1015 15th St. NW
Washington DC 20005

American Red Cross
17th and D Streets NW
Washington D.C. 20006

American School Health
Association
P.O. Box 708
1521 South Water Street
Kent OH 44240

American Society of
Childbirth
P.O. Box 16159
7113 Lynnwood Drive
Tampa FL 33687

American Urological
Association Allied
6845 Lake Shore Drive
P.O. Box 9397
Raytown MO 64133

Association of the Care of
Children in Hospitals
3615 Wisconsin Avenue NW
Washington D.C. 20016

International Committee of
Catholic Nurses & Social
Assistants
Palazzo S. Calisto
1-00120 Cittadel Vaticano
Italy

International Council of Nurses
3 Place Jean Marteau
1201 Geneva
Switzerland

Joint Commission on Accreditation of Hospitals
875 North Michigan Ave.
Chicago IL 60611

Mid-Atlantic Regional Nursing Organization
Teachers College - Columbia University
Box 146
525 W. 120th St.
New York NY 10027

Midwest Alliance in Nursing
Indiana University
1226 W. Michigan Street
Room 108-BR
Indianapolis IN 46223

National Institutes of Health
900 Rockville Pike
Bethesda MD 20205

National Kidney Association
2 Park Avenue
New York NY 10016

National League of Nursing
10 Columbus Circle
New York NY 10019-1350

National Student Nurses' Association
10 Columbus Circle
New York NY 10019-1350

New England Organization of Nursing
55 Chapel Street
Newton MA 02160

Office of Human Development Service
Office of Policy and Legislation
200 Independence Avenue SW
Washington DC 20201

Pan American Health Organization
525 23rd Street NW
Washington DC 20037

Peace Corps
806 Connecticut Avenue NW Rm. P-301
Washington DC 20526

People to People Health
Foundation (Project
HOPE)
Millwood VA 22646

Sigma Theta Tau National
Honor Society of
Nursing
1100 Waterway Boulevard
Indianapolis IN 46202

Southern Council of
Collegiate Education for
Nursing
1340 Spring Street NW
Atlanta GA 30309

U.S. Office of Personnel
Management
1900 E Street NW
Washington D.C. 20415

U.S. Public Health Service
Dept. of Health & Human
Services
5600 Fishers Lane
Rockville MD 20857

Western Interstate
Commission for Higher
Education
P.O. Drawer P
Boulder CO 80302

World Federation of
Neurosurgical Nurses
286 W. 2nd Street
Morristown NJ 08057

World Health Organization
Avenue Appia 1211
Geneva 27
Switzerland

APPENDIX E

State Nurses Associations

Alabama State Nurses Association
Montgomery
(205) 262-8321

Alaska Nurses Association
Anchorage
(907) 274-0827

Arizona Nurses Association
Tempe
(602) 831-0404

California Nurses Association
San Francisco
(415) 864-4141

Colorado Nurses Association
Denver
(303) 757-7484

Connecticut Nurses Association
Meridan
(203) 238-1207

Delaware Nurses Association
Newark
(302) 368-2333

District of Columbia Nurses Association, Inc.
Washington DC
(202) 244-2705

Florida Nurses Association
Orlando
(407) 896-3261

Georgia Nurses Association Inc.
Atlanta
(404) 876-4624

Guam Nurses Association
Agana Guam
(617) 734-9162

Hawaii Nurses Association
Honolulu
(808) 531-1628/521-8361

Idaho Nurses Association
Boise
(208) 345-0500

Illinois Nurses Association
Chicago
(312) 236-9708

Indiana State Nurses Association
Indianapolis
(317) 299-4575/4576

Iowa Nurses Association
Des Moines
(515) 282-9169

Kansas State Nurses Association
Topeka
(913) 233-8638

Kentucky Nurses Association
Louisville
(502) 637-2546/2547

Louisiana State Nurses Association
Metairie
(504) 889-1030

Maine State Nurses Association
Augusta
(207) 622-1057

Maryland Nurses Association, Inc.
Baltimore
(301) 242-7300

Massachusetts Nurses Association
Canton
(617) 821-4625

Michigan Nurses Association
Okemos
(517) 349-5640

Minnesota Nurses Association
St. Paul
(612) 646-4807/0927

Mississippi Nurses Association
Jackson
(601) 982-9182/9183

Missouri Nurses Association
Jefferson City
(314) 636-4623

Montana Nurses Association
Helena
(406) 442-6710

Nebraska Nurses Association
Lincoln
(402) 475-3859

Nevada Nurses Association
Reno
(702) 825-3555

New Hampshire Nurses Association
Concord
(603) 225-3783

New Jersey State Nurses Association
Trenton
(609) 392-4884/2031

New Mexico Nurses Association
Albuquerque
(505) 268-7744

New York State Nurses Association
Guilderland
(518) 456-5371

North Carolina Nurses Association
Raleigh
(919) 821-4250

North Dakota Nurses Association
Bismarck
(701) 223-1385

Ohio Nurses Association
Columbus
(614) 237-5414

Oklahoma Nurses Association
Oklahoma City
(405) 840-3476

Oregon Nurses Association, Inc.
Portland
(503) 293-0011

Pennsylvania Nurses Association
Harrisburg
(717) 657-1222

Rhode Island State Nurses Association
Providence
(401) 421-9703

South Carolina Nurses Association
Columbia
(803) 252-4781

South Dakota Nurses Association, Inc.
Sioux Falls
(605) 338-1401

Tennessee Nurses Association
Nashville
(615) 254-0350

Texas Nurses Association
Austin
(512) 452-0645

Utah Nurses Association
Salt Lake City
(801) 322-3439

Vermont State Nurses Association, Inc.
South Burlington
(802) 864-9390

Virgin Islands Nurses Association
Christiansted
St. Croix U.S. Virgin Islands
(809) 773-2323 Ext. 116/154

Virginia Nurses Association
Richmond
(804) 353-7311

Washington State Nurses Association
Seattle
(206) 443-9762

West Virginia Nurses Association, Inc.
Charleston
(304) 342-1169

Wisconsin Nurses Association, Inc.
Madison
(608) 221-0383

Wyoming Nurses
Association
Cheyenne
(307) 635-3955

APPENDIX F

Nursing Specialty Organizations

Aerospace Medical
Association
Flight Nurse—Section ASMA
PSC Box 3009
APO NY 09223

American Academy of
Ambulatory Nursing
Administration
N. Woodbury Rd.
Box 56
Pittman NJ 08071

American Assembly for Men
in Nursing
c/o College of Nursing
Rush University
600 S. Paulina—474-H
Chicago Il 60612

American Association for
Critical Care Nurses
One Civic Plaza
Newport Beach CA 92660

American Association of
Industrial Nurses
P.O. Box 478
Dallas TX 75221

American Association of
Nephrology Nurses
N. Woodbury Rd.
Box 56
Pittman NJ 08071

American Association of
NeuroScience Nurses
22 S. Washington St. Ste. 203
Park Ridge IL 60068

American Association of
Neurosurgical Nurses
625 N. Michigan Ave.
Ste. 1519
Chicago IL 60611

American Association of
Nurse Anesthetists
216 Higgins Rd.
Park Ridge IL 60068

American Association of
Nurse Attorneys
P.O. Box 5564
Washington D.C. 20005

American Association of
Occupational Health
Nurses
3500 Piedmont Rd. NE
Atlanta GA 30305

American College of Nurse-
Midwives
1522 K St. NW, Suite 1120
Washington D.C. 20005

American Holistic Nurses'
Association
P.O. Box 116
Telluride CO 81435

American Indian/Alaska
Native
Nurses' Association, Inc.
P.O. Box 1588
Norman OK 73070

American Society of
Ophthalmic Registered
Nurses, Inc.
P.O. Box 3030
San Francisco CA 94119

American Society of Plastic
& Reconstructive
Surgical Nurses
N. Woodbury Rd.
Box 56
Pittman NJ 08071

American Society of Post-
Anesthesia Nurses
2315 Westwood Ave., Ste. 1
P.O. Box 11083
Richmond VA 23230

Association for Practitioners
in Infection Control
505 E. Hawley St.
Mundelein IL 60060

Association of Nurses
Practicing Independently
21 Spruce St.
Dept. NL
Dansville NY 14437

Association of Operating
Room Nurses
10170 E. Mississippi Ave.
Denver CO 80231

Association of Pediatric/
Oncology Nurses
Pacific Medical Center
P.O. Box 7999
San Francisco CA 94120

Association of Rehabilitation
Nurses
2506 Gross Point Rd.
Evanston IL 60201

Commission on Graduates
of Foreign Nursing
Schools
3624 Market St.
Philadelphia PA 19104

Dermatology Nurses'
Association
N. Woodbury Rd.
Box 56
Pittman NJ 08071

Emergency Nurses'
Association
666 North Lake Shore Drive
Suite 1131
Chicago IL 60611

Gerontological Nursing
844 West End
Annapolis MD 21401

International Association for
Enterstomal Therapy, Inc.
One Newport Place
Suite 970
Newport Beach CA 92660

Lesbian & Gay Nurses'
Alliance
801 E. Harrison Ste. 105
Seattle WA 98102

National Association for
Health Care Recruitment
P.O. Box 93851
Cleveland OH 44101

National Association for
Practical Nurse Education
& Service
10801 Pear Tree Lane
Suite 151
St. Louis MO 63134

National Association of
Hispanic Nurses
2014 Johnston St.
Los Angeles CA 90031

National Association of
Nurse Recruiters
30 Woodland Drive.
Churchville PA 18966

National Association of
Orthopaedic Nurses
N. Woodbury Rd.
Box 56
Pittman NJ 08071

National Association of
Pediatric Nurse
Associates &
Practitioners
1000 Maplewood Dr.
Ste. 104
Maple Shade NJ 08052

National Association of
Physician's Nurses
9401 Lee Hwy. Suite 210
Fairfax VA 22031

National Association of
Quality Assurance
Professionals Inc.
Dept. NL
1800 Pickwick Ave.
Glenview IL 60025

National Association of
School Nurses Inc.
P.O. Box 1300
Lamplighter Lane
Scarborough ME 04074

National Black Nurses'
Association Inc.
P.O. Box 18358
Boston MA 02118

National Flight Nurses'
Association
Life Flight
Allegheny General Hospital
320 E. North Ave.
Pittsburg PA 15212

National Intravenous
Therapy Association, Inc.
87 Blanchard Rd.
Cambridge MA 02138

National Nurses' Society on Addictions
2506 Gross Point Rd.
Evanston IL 60201

National Nurses' Society on Alcoholism
P.O. Box 7728
Indian Creek Branch
Shawnee Mission KS 66207

Nurses' Alliance for the Prevention of Nuclear War
Box 319
Chestnut Hill MA 02167

Nurses' Association of the American College of Obstetrics & Gynecologists
600 Maryland Ave. SW
Suite 200 East
Washington D.C. 20024

Nurses' Christian Fellowship
233 Langdon St.
Madison WI 53703

Nurses' Coalition for Action in Politics
1030 15th St. NW Suite 408
Washington D.C. 20005

Nurse Consultants' Association
P.O. Box 25875
Colorado Springs CO 80936

Nurses' Educational Funds Inc.
555 W. 57th Street
New York NY 10019

Nurses' House Inc.
10 Columbus Circle
New York NY 10019

Nurses in Transition
P.O. Box 14472
San Francisco CA 94114

Nurses Now
P.O. Box 5156
Pittsburgh PA 15206

Oncology Nursing Society
3111 Banksville Rd.
Pittsburgh PA 15216

Otolaryngology & Head/
Neck Nurses
c/o Warren Otologic Group
3893 E. Market Street
Warren OH 44484

Public Health Nursing/
American Public Health
Association
1015 Fifteenth St. NW
Washington D.C. 20005

Society for Advancement in
Nursing Inc.
Cooper Station Box 307
11th St. & 4th Ave.
New York NY 10003

Society for Parenteral &
External Nutrition
1025 Vermont Ave. NW
Suite 8110-Dept. N 81
Washington D.C. 20005

Society for Peripheral
Vascular Nursing
1070 Sibley Tower
Rochester NY 14604

Society for Research in
Nursing Education
School of Nursing N319Y
UCSF
Third & Parnassus Ave.
San Francisco CA 94143

The Society for Nursing
History
Nursing Education
Department
Box 150
Teachers College
Columbia University
New York NY 10027

Transcultural Nursing
Society
College of Nursing
University of Utah
25 S. Medical Drive
Salt Lake City UT 84112

United Nurses' Associations
of California
170 W San Jose Ave. Ste. 102
Claremont CA 91711

United Nursing Home
Association
16400 Southcenter Prkwy.
Suite 410
Seattle WA 98188

APPENDIX G

Nursing/Medical Organizations

The following organizations provide support and information for nurses in the United States.

American Nurses Association—ANA

Since its inception in 1896, ANA has focused on fostering high standards of nursing practice, promoting the welfare of practitioners, and improving the general working conditions of nurses. ANA has served as the only full-service professional organization for the nation's entire registered nurse population.

ANA establishes and implements nursing's political and legislative programs, fosters a professional and equitable work enviornment for all nurses, and develops standards that ensure high quality patient care in institutions and the community.

More than 200,000 registered nurses are represented in ANA through its 52 State Nursing Associations. When nurses join their state nurses association, they automatically gain benefits of membership in ANA. Through ANA, members can participate in a variety of programs, ranging from economic and general welfare to financial planning and support and information networks, that enable nurses to work more effectively with their employers, resolve legal and ethical concerns, and practice nursing according to the highest standards.

ANA publishes the *American Journal of Nursing (AJN)* each month. The journal provides information on current issues, problems, concerns, and treatments in nursing practice.

For further information, contact:

ANA Communications Unit
600 Maryland Ave., SW
Suite 100W
Washington, DC 20024-2571
Tel: (202) 554-4444, ext. 247

National League for Nursing

The National League for Nursing (NLN) seeks to identify the nursing needs of society and foster programs designed to meet these needs. The League also develops and supports services for the improvement of nursing service and nursing education through consultation, continuing education, testing, accreditation, evaluation, and other activities.

NLN works with voluntary, governmental and other agencies, groups, and organizations for the advancement of nursing and toward the achievement of comprehensive health care.

NLN publishes a journal as well as fourteen different newsletters that target nursing practice and education, assessment, health care policy, etc. The League also boasts of an abundance of timely books and videos that are available to members at a discount.

Additional benefits include networking opportunities, reduced-rate group insurance programs, and NLN Gold Mastercard Program.

Membership fees are contingent upon the category selected. Further information about NLN may be obtained by contacting:

National League for Nursing
350 Hudson Street
New York, NY 10014-4504
Tel: 1-800-669-1656

The following organizations offer support, networking, and business expertise for nurses who opt for nontraditional nursing opportunities. The information provided has been condensed from documentation received from the various organizations. The intent is to present an objective picture of each organization that allows the reader to determine whether or not a particular association has something to offer him or her.

National Nurses in Business Association

The National Nurses in Business Association (NNBA) is dedicated to expanding the role of nurses in business by:

(1) Promoting nurse entrepreneurs and nurse intrapreneurs to develop, grow, own or manage businesses within the health care industry.

(2) Developing opportunities locally and nationally for nurses in business.

(3) Serving the networking and educational needs of members.

NNBA's mission is to integrate the art of nursing and the world of business in order to help nurses reach their personal career goals and, concurrently, to elevate awareness of the uniqueness of nurses and the business of health care.

Membership in NNBA is extremely helpful for the individual who:

- wishes to explore health care business career options
- wants to start his/her own nursing business
- already operates an existing healthcare business
- is working for a company involved in any aspect of health care (service or product)

Individual memberships are $95.00/year. For additional information about NNBA write or call:

National Nurses in Business Association
1000 Burnett Avenue, Suite 450
Concord, CA 94520
Tel: (510) 356-2642 or
FAX: (510) 356-2654

Alliance for Health Care Strategy and Marketing

The Alliance provides the health care industry with education and information on current strategies for business growth and the tools for successful implementation. It is an international membership organization for healthcare professionals involved in the strategic leadership of their organizations to ensure market responsiveness. Members of Alliance join a unique network of executives from across the health care industry: integrated delivery systems, managed care, hospitals, medical group practices, home healthcare, ambulatory care, academic medical centers, and others.

This executive network includes strategy and marketing professionals, chief executive officers managed care professionals, clinicians, physicians, quality directors, and managers of specialty care. Membership dues are $125 annually. For more information, contact:

Alliance for Healthcare Strategy and Marketing
11 South LaSalle Street,
Suite 2300
Chicago, IL 60603
Tel: (312) 704-9700 or
FAX: (312) 704-9709

American Medical Writers Association

The objectives of AMWA are to bring together into one association individuals who are interested in any aspect of communication in the medical and allied scientific professions. The organization also seeks to promote standards of excellence in biomedical communications as well as to inform and encourage all those interested in improving the quality and effectiveness of biomedical communications. Finally, AMWA provides educational opportunities that lead to, support, and enhance excellence in medical communication.

The organization holds an annual conference which offers four days of workshops, plenary sessions, seminars, tours, and networking opportunities. Regional meetings with workshops are held throughout the year. There are also local chapter meetings and book award competitions and journalism awards.

Benefits of membership include: job market publications for employment opportunities, membership and freelance directories, core curriculum programs which offer certificates upon completion, etc.

Annual dues are $75.00. For additional information contact:

American Medical Writers
Association
9650 Rockville Pike
Bethesda, MD 20814
Tel: (301) 493-0003
FAX: (301)493-0005

American Association of Legal Nurse Consultants

The AALNC was formed in July 1989 as a professional association for Registered Nurses consulting in the legal field. The purpose of the AALNC is to promote professional advancement for RNs who are actively practicing in a consulting capacity to the legal profession and to provide a resource for information on matters relating to legal aspects of nursing and health care law.

Benefits and privileges of the organization include:

- Access to a national network of over 1,300 members and to local chartered chapters nationwide.
- Quarterly publication, *NETWORK*, providing up-to-date information on medical, legal, and consultant practice issues, case law updates and employment opportunities.

- Malpractice insurance, with reasonable premiums, designed for AALNC members by Macginnis & Associates.
- Membership directory published annually, with cross-indexing, including identification of nurse experts and nurse consultants in each geographic area.
- Educational opportunities (national conferences, regional seminars and chapter leadership forums).
- Opportunity to network with professionals in related fields including attorneys, paralegals, legal assistants, physicians, and other specialists.
- Latest information on medical-legal issues and practice as a legal nurse consultant.

Membership is available in three categories: Active ($85.00), Associate ($85.00), Sustaining ($150.00). For further information, contact:

American Association of Legal Nurse
Consultants
500 North Michigan Avenue, Suite 1400
Chicago, IL 60611
Tel: (312) 670-0550
FAX: (312) 661-0769

National Association for Quality Assurance

This association was founded in 1976 and has more than 6,500 members. It is dedicated to promoting quality health care for all patients and is the primary educational source for quality management professionals.

Membership is open to the individual who specializes in quality management. This includes quality improvement, utilization management, risk management, discharge planning/ continuity of care, infection control, etc.

The association sends out a bimonthly publication, *Journal for Healthcare Quality*, to all members. A regional newsletter is published quarterly, which provides pertinent news and information at the local/regional level. An educational conference which offers opportunities to meet with other members and exchange ideas and information is held each year. A membership directory, published annually, is available to members only and is invaluable as a resource tool.

In addition, members benefit from formal liaisons with other organizations such as the American Hospital Association, Joint Commission on Accreditation of Healthcare Organizations (JCAHO), National Health Council. NAHQ also has working relationships with several other groups, including the American Nurses Association.

Further information may be obtained by contacting:

National Association for
Healthcare Quality
5700 Old Orchard Road,
First Floor
Skokie, IL 60077-1057
Tel: (708) 966-9392
FAX: (708) 966-9418

American Society for Health Care Marketing & Public Relations

This is an organization of more than 3,000 professionals who manage marketing, public relations, public affairs, and related disciplines. As the only society dedicated exclusively to health care marketing and public relations professionals,

ASHCMPR is committed to providing the most comprehensive and useful services to help members and their organizations succeed.

The Society sponsors the profession's premier educational conference and trade show exhibition, in addition to in-depth seminars and workshops throughout the year.

Members stay abreast of new programs and trends with the Society's newsletter *Health Care Marketing and Public Relations*, which alternates every other month with *The Resource Collection*, a compendium of successful case studies and timely reference materials.

The society offers an annual Membership Directory as well as a *Directory of Health Care Marketing, Planning, and Public Relations Consultants.*

Depending on category, annual membership fees range from $75.00 (student) to $280.00 (joint associate). Additional information may be obtained from:

American Society for Health Care Marketing & Public Relations
of the American Hospital Association
840 North Lake Shore Drive
Chicago, IL 60611
Tel: (312) 280-6359

APPENDIX H

Magazines And Journals

More than 120 journals and magazines are published for, on, or about nursing each year. Some of these are published in the United States. Others in Europe, Canada, Australia, etc. All are available to nurses in the United States.

Many of these publications offer hands-on information about nursing skills, techniques, etc., while others are more intellectual in nature and deal with studies and research.

AANA Journal: American Association of Nurse Anesthetists Journal

AACN: Clinical Issues in Critical Care Nursing

AAOHN: American Association of Occupational Health Nursing

Advances in Nursing Science: $64 per year.

Contact: Advances in Nursing Science, Aspen Publishers, Inc., 7201 McKinney Circle, Frederick MD 21701.

AIDS Patient Care: $89 per year. Checks payable to Liebert Publications, Inc.

Contact: Mary Ann Liebert, Inc., 1651 Third Avenue, New York, NY 10128-3649.

American Journal of Hospice & Palliative Care: $66 per year.

Contact: The American Journal of Hospice & Palliative Care, 470 Boston Post Road, Weston, MA 02193-9943.

AJN: American Journal of Nursing. AJN offers a thorough compilation of information on general nursing procedures. It might be regarded as the "update bible" for floor/ward nurses. $22.97 per year.

Contact: American Journal of Nursing, P.O. Box 50478, Boulder, CO 80321-0478.

AORN: Association of Operating Room Nurses journal. Available automatically to members of AORN. Provides insight and information regarding situations and new technologies in the perioperative setting.

Contact: AORN Journal, 2170 S. Parker Road, Suite 300, Denver, CO 80231-5711.

Archives of Psychiatric Nursing: $44 per year.

Contact: Archives of Psychiatric Nursing, Periodicals Order Fulfillment Department, W.B. Saunders Company, 6277 Sea Harbor Drive, Orlando, FL 32821-9989.

Cancer Nursing—An International Journal for Cancer Care: $44 per year.

Contact: Raven Press, Subscription Department, 1185 Avenue of the Americas, 37th Floor, New York, NY 10109-0403.

Caring: Published by the National Association for Home Care. $45 per year.

Contact: Caring, National Association for Home Care, 519 C Street, N.E., Washington, DC, 20077-0646.

Clinical Nurse Specialist: Covers the roles of the clinical nurse specialist as clinician, researcher, consultant, executive, peer and patient educator—regardless of specialty. $67 per year.

Contact: Williams & Wilkins, P.O. Box 23291, Baltimore, MD 21298-9325.

Clinics in Geriatric Nursing

Computers in Nursing: $50 per year.

Contact: J. B. Lippincott, P.O. Box 1600, Hagerstown, MD 21741-9932.

Critical Care Nurse: $27 per year.

Contact: Critical Care Nurse, P.O.Box 611, Holmes, PA 19043-9873.

Critical Care Nursing Clinics of North America

Critical Care Nursing Quarterly: Provides information on such issues as unit design, advances in neurosciences, multi-systems crisis, cardiomyopathy. $63 per year.

Contact: Aspen Publishers, P.O. Box 990, Frederick, MD 21705-9782.

Dermatology Nursing: $28 per year.

Contact: Dermatology Nursing, Jannetti Publications, Inc., East Holly Avenue, Box 56, Pitman, NJ 08071-9911.

Gastroenterology Nursing: Official journal of the Society of GE nurses and assistants. Members of SGNA receive the magazine as part of their membership. Non-members pay $63 per year.

Contact: Gastroenterology Nursing, 428 E. Preston Street, Baltimore, MD 21203-3993.

Geriatric Nursing: A source for clinical information and management advice relevant to the care of older adults in all settings. $29 per year.

Contact: Geriatric Nursing, Journal Subscription Services, Mosby-Year Book, Inc.11830 Westline Industrial Drive, St. Louis, MO 63146-9988.

Health Care Supervisor

Heart & Lung: The Journal of Critical Care: Presents information on techniques, advances, investigations, and observations concerning the care of critically ill patients. $36 per year.

Contact: Heart & Lung: The Journal of Critical Care, Journal Subscription Services, Mosby—Year Book, Inc., 11830 Westline Industrial Drive, St. Louis, MO 63146-9988.

Holistic Nursing Practice: A peer-reviewed journal that provides nurse clinicians and educators with information on holistic approaches to nursing practice in clinical settings. Provides articles on such topics as Health, Risk and Nursing Practice, Collaboration in the Acute Care Setting, Women's Health, Leadership in Nursing. $71 per year.

Contact: Holistic Nursing Practice, Aspen Publishers, P.O. Box 990, Frederick, MD 21705-9782.

Home Health Care Services Quarterly

Home Health Care Nurse: $36 per year.

Contact: Home Health Care Nurse, J.B. Lippincott, P.O. Box 1600, Hagerstown, MD 21741-9932.

IMAGE: The Journal of Nursing Scholarship: The official journal of Sigma Theta Tau International Honor Society for Nursing, Inc. $16 per year.

Contact: IMAGE Publication Office, Sigma Theta Tau International Society for Nursing, Inc. 550 West North Street, Indianapolis, IN 46202.

Intensive & Critical Care Nursing: The aim of I & CCN is: to promote excellence in the care of the critically ill patient by specialist nurses and their professional colleagues; to provide an international and interdisciplinary forum for the publication, dissemination and exchange of research findings, experience, and ideas; to develop and enhance the knowledge, skills, attitudes, and creative thinking essential to good critical care nursing practice. $112 per year.

Contact: Intensive and Critical Care Nursing, Sales Promotion Department, Churchill Livingstone Journals, Robert Stevenson House, 1-3 Baxter's Place, Edinburgh, EH1 3AF, UK.

International Journal of Health Services

International Journal of Nursing Studies

International Nursing Review

Issues in Comprehensive Pediatric Nursing

The Joint Commission Journal on Quality Improvement: Provides practical tools to improve quality in health care. The Journal publishes original manuscripts on innovative thinking, strategies, and practices in measuring, assessing, and improving performance in health care. $115 per year

Contact: The Joint Commission Journal on Quality Improvement, Journal Subscription Services, Mosby-Year Book, Inc. 11830 Westline Industrial Drive, St. Louis MO 63146-9988.

Journal of Ambulatory Care Management: Offers the latest information on professional liability, Medicaid coverage, financial management, computerized patient tracking blood donors, AIDS, etc. $105 per year.

Contact: The Journal of Ambulatory Care Management, Aspen Publishers, P.O. Box 990, Frederick, MD 21705-9782.

Journal of Cardiovascular Nursing: Offers such topical articles as Mechanical Interventions for the Failing Heart, Social Support: Helpful or Harmful, Changing Paradigms for Understanding Cardiovascular Disorders, Cardiovascular Risk Factor Modification. $64 per year.

Contact: Journal of Cardiovascular Nursing, Aspen Publishers, P.O. Box 990, Frederick, MD 21705-9782.

Journal of Community Health Nursing

Journal of Continuing Education in Nursing

Journal of Emergency Nursing: $44 per year.

Contact: Journal of Emergency Nursing, Journal Subscription Services, Mosby—Year Book, Inc., 11830 Westline Industrial Drive, St. Louis, MO 63146-9988.

Journal of Enterstomal Therapy

Journal of Gerontological Nursing

Journal of Holistic Nursing

Journal of Home Health Care Practice: Recent issues discussed include Managed Care: Our Changing Industry, Aging, Management/Clinical Expertise, Home Infusion Therapy. $64 per year.

Contact: Journal of Home Health Care Practice, Aspen Publishers, P.O. Box 990, Frederick, MD 21705-9782.

Journal of Intravenous Nursing: $60 per year.

Contact: Journal of Intravenous Nursing, J. B.Lippincott, P.O. Box 1600, Hagerstown, MD 21741-9932.

Journal of Neuroscience Nursing

Journal of Nurse-Midwifery

Journal of Nursing Administration: $60 per year.

Contact: Journal of Nursing Administration, J.B. Lippincott, P.O. Box 1600, Hagerstown, MD 21741-9932.

Journal of Nursing Care Quality: A sample of recent articles includes: Quality Improvement: Programs and Methods, Using Data to Improve Quality, Effective Quality Teams, Process Improvement. $77 per year.

Contact: Journal of Nursing Care Quality, Aspen Publishers, P.O. Box 990, Frederick, MD 21705-9782.

Journal of Nursing Education

Journal of Nursing Measurement: The primary focus of the Journal is the development and testing of instruments for measuring the effectiveness of nursing procedures, as well as evidence for the reliability, validity, sensitivity, or specificity of these instruments. In addition, there are discussions of innovative theories, principles, practices, and issues relevant to nursing measurement. $29 per year.

Contact: Journal of Nursing Measurement, Springer Publishing Company, 536 Broadway, New York, NY 10012.

Journal of Nursing Staff Development: $54 per year.

Contact: Journal of Nursing Staff Development, J. B. Lippincott, P.O. Box 1600, Hagerstown, MD 21741-9932.

Journal of Obstetric, Gynecologic, and Neonatal Nursing: $55 per year.

Contact: Journal of Obstetric, Gynecologic, and Neonatal Nursing, J. B. Lippincott, P.O. Box 1600, Hagerstown, MD 21741-9932.

Journal of Ophthalmic Nursing & Technology

Contact: Journal of Ophthalmic Nursing & Technology, 6900 Grove Road, Thorofare, NJ 08086.

Journal of Pediatric Nursing

Journal of Pediatric Oncology Nursing: Official journal of the Association of Pediatric Oncology Nurses. $49 per year.

Contact: Journal of Pediatric Oncology Nursing, Periodicals Order Fulfillment Department, W. B. Saunders Company, 6277 Sea Harbor Drive, Orlando, FL 32821-9989.

Journal of Perinatology: $50 per year.

Contact: Journal of Perinatology, Journal Subscription Services, Mosby-Year Book, Inc., 11830 Westline Industrial Drive, St. Louis, MO 63146-9988.

Journal of Post Ansesthesia Nursing: $56 per year.

Contact: Journal of Post Anesthesia Nursing, Periodical Orders Fulfillment, W. B. Saunders Company, 6277 Sea Harbor Drive, Orlando, FL 32821-9989.

Journal of Prison & Jail Health

Journal of Professional Nursing: $64 per year.

Contact: Journal of Professional Nursing, W. B. Saunders Company, 6277 Sea Harbor Drive, Orlando, FL 32821-9989.

Journal of Psychosocial Nursing and Mental Health Services: $48 per year.

Contact: Journal of Psychosocial Nursing and Mental Health Services, 6900 Grove Road, Thorofare, NJ 08086-9864.

Journal of School Nursing

Journal of the American Academy of Nurse Practitioners

Journal of Transcultural Nursing

Journal of Urological Nursing

Journal of Wound, Ostomy & Continence Nursing: $46 per year.

Contact: Journal of Wound, Ostomy & Continence Nursing, Journal Subscription Services, Mosby-Year Book, Inc., 11830 Westline Industrial Drive, St. Louis, MO 63146-9988.

MCN: Maternal Child Nursing Journal: $21.97 per year.

Contact: MCN Subscription, P.O.Box 53435, Boulder, CO 80321-3435.

Midwives Chronicle

National Black Nurses' Association Journal

Nurse Education Today—An International Journal: $136 per year.

Contact Churchill Livingstone Journals, Subscription Department, Longman Group Ltd., P.O. Box 77, Hanlow, Essex CM 19 5 BQ.

Nurse Educator: $45 per year.

Contact: Nurse Educator, J. B. Lippincott, P.O. Box 1600, Hagerstown, MD 21741-9932.

Nurse Practitioner: $42 per year.

Contact: The Nurse Practitioner, P.O. Box 882, New York, NY 10160-0206.

Nursing '95: $42 per year.

Contact: Nursing '95, One Health Care Drive, P.O. Box 2021, Marion, OH 43306-2121.

Nursing Administrative Quarterly

Nursing Economic$: $30 per year.

Contact: Nursing Economic$, Jannetti Publications, Inc., East Holly Avenue, Box 56, Pitman, NJ 08071-9911.

Nursing & Health Care: $40 per year.

Contact: Nursing & Health Care, National League for Nursing, 350 Hudson Street, New York, NY 10014-9899.

Nursing Forum

Nursing Management: $32 per year.

Contact: Nursing Management, 434 W. Downer Place, Aurora, IL 60506-9633.

Nursing Outlook: $31 per year.

Contact: Nursing Outlook, Journal Subscription Services, Mosby-Year Book, Inc., 11830 Westline Industrial Drive, St. Louis, MO 63146-9988.

Nursing Research: The research journal of the American Nurses Association. $40 per year.

Contact: Nursing Research, P.O. Box 58766, Boulder, CO 80321-8766.

Nursing Science Quarterly: Deals with theory, research and practice. $50 per year.

Contact: Nursing Science Quarterly, Chestnut House Publications, P.O. Box 22492, Pittsburgh, PA 15222-0492.

Nursing Times: An English publication.

Contact: Nursing Times Reader Department, 2 Ridgeway Road, Farnham, Surrey GU9 8NW.

ORL—Head & Neck Nursing

Orthopedic Nursing: The journal for the National Association of Orthopedic Nurses. $21 per year, if check enclosed; $24 per year, when billed later.

Contact: Orthopedic Nursing, c/o Anthony J. Jannetti, Inc., East Holly Avenue, Box 56, Pitman, NJ 08071-0056.

Patient Care

Pediatric Nursing: $21 per year, if check enclosed; $24 per year, when billed later.

Contact: Pediatric Nursing, Anthony J. Jannetti, Inc., East Holly Avenue, Box 56, Pitman, NJ 08071-9911.

Public Health Nursing: $52 per year.

Contact: Public Health Nursing, Blackwell Scientific Publications, Inc., 238 Main Street, Cambridge, MA 02142.

Rehabilitation Nursing

Research in Nursing & Health

Revolution—The Journal of Nurse Empowerment: Takes on the more controversial issues that plague nurses like floating, doctor/nurse confrontations, sexual harassment; discusses them and offers solutions and/or options. It also features timely articles about healthcare reform, hospital restructuring, and alternatives to traditional nursing jobs or careers. $24.95 per year.

Contact: Revolution—The Journal of Nurse Empowerment, A.D. Von Publishers, Inc., 56 McArthur Avenue, Staten Island, NY 10312.

RN: $35 per year.

Contact: RN, Circulation Department, P.O. Box 57140, Boulder, CO 80322-7140.

Scholarly Inquiry for Nursing Practice: International in scope and crosses traditional disciplinary lines to draw upon theory and methodology from other fields. Papers include quantitative research, both basic and applied, state-of-the-art reviews, and theory-based tool development. In this format, authors and noted commentators together move through the inquiry process to test new and evolving ideas and to explore how they relate to clinical interventions. $42.00 per year.

Contact: Scholarly Inquiry for Nursing Practice, Springer Publishing Company, 536 Broadway, New York, NY 10012.

APPENDIX I

References

"Acute Care NPs Chart a New Career Path for Hospital RNs." *American Journal of Nursing*, June 1994, 94(6): 69-73.

Aiken, Linda H., RN, PhD, and Mullinix, Connie Flint, RN, MPH, MBA. "The Nursing Shortage: Myth or Reality?" *The New England Journal of Medicine*, September 3, 1987, 317(10): 641-645.

Aiken, T. D. "Lobbying and What Nurses Can do to Promote Legislation." *AORN Journal*, August 1991, 54(2): 220-1, 223.

Allen, Teresa, RN, Brady, Joan, RN, and Vonfrolio, Laura G., RN. *25 Stupid Things Nurses Do To Self Destruct.* New York: Power Publications, 1995.

"ANA Delegates Act to Prepare Nurses for Their Future." *American Journal of Nursing*, August 1993, 93(8): 71-73.

Anders, George. "Nurses Decry Cost-Cutting Plan That Uses Aides to Do More Jobs." *Wall Street Journal*, January 24, 1994, p. B1.

Aydelotte, Myrtle K. "Nursing's Preferred Future." *Nursing Outlook*, May/June 1987, 35(3):114-120.

Baer, Ellen D. "The Feminist Disdain for Nursing." *The New York Times*, February 23, 1991, p. 24.

Barkley, Thomas W., Jr., RN, MSN, and Kohler, Patricia A., RN, MS, MSN. "Is Nursing's Image a Deterrent to Recruiting Men into the Profession? Male High School Students Respond." *Nursing Forum*, April-June 1992, 28(2): 9-14.

Batra, Carol, RN, PhD. "Empowering for Professional, Political, and Health Policy Involvement." *Nursing Outlook*, July/August 1992 40(4): 170-176.

Berg, Elizabeth. "The Crisis Nobody Talks About: Where Are the Nurses?" *Woman's Day*, Jan. 7, 1992, (2): 54.

Blenkarn, Helen, D'Amico, Mary, and Virtue, Elaine. "Primary Nursing and Job Satisfaction." *Nursing Management*, April 1988, 19(4): 41-42.

"Boston, Chicago RNs Rally to Fight New Invasions of Unlicensed Workers." *American Journal of Nursing*, August 1993, 93(8): 70.

Bowman, Ann Marie, RN, MS. "Victim Blaming in Nursing." *Nursing Outlook*, November/December 1993, 41(6): 268-273.

Brady, Joan. "Nurses—An Endangered Species." *Revolution: The Journal of Nursing Empowerment*, Spring 1995: 10-12.

__________. "Putting Out Fires" *Revolution: The Journal of Nursing Empowerment*, Summer 1994: 38-39.

Braun, Kathryn, Christle, Donna, Walker, Duane, and Tiwanek, Gail. "Verbal Abuse of Nurses and Non-Nurses."

Nursing Management, March 1991, 22(3): 72-76.

"BSN Schools See Graduations Gaining, More Men Choosing Nursing Careers." *American Journal of Nursing*, June 1992, 92(6): 84, 88.

Burda, David. "Tough Road Ahead for Nurse Panel." *Modern Healthcare*, July 18, 1994, 24(29): 18-19.

Buresh, Bernice. "Nursing Goes Public." *Revolution: The Journal of Nursing Empowerment*, Spring 1995: 16-20.

__________. "Television Coverage of Healthcare—Can Nurses Break In?" *Revolution: The Journal of Nursing Empowerment*, Summer 1993:14-16, 104-105.

Buresh, Bernice, Gordon, Suzanne, and Bell, Nica. "Who Counts in News Coverage of Health Care?" *Nursing Outlook*, September/October 1991, 39(5): 204-208.

Califano, Joseph A., Jr. "The Nurse as a Revolutionary." *Revolution: The Journal of Nursing Empowerment*, Fall 1993: 66-68, 108-110.

"California RNs Attack Work Redesign as Patient 'Fraud'." *American Journal of Nursing*, November 1994, 94(11): 69.

"Caring is Not Enough for a Career." *The Economist*, January 16, 1988, p. 49.

Carlson-Catalano, Judy, EdD, RN. "Empowering Nurses for Professional Practice." *Nursing Outlook*, May/June 1992, 40(3): 139-142.

Chandler, G. E. "Nurses in the News: From Invisible to Visible." *Journal of Nursing Administration*, February 1992, 22(2): 11-12.

Chinn, P. L. "Where and When Does Change Begin?" (editorial), *Nursing Outlook*, May/June 1992, 40(3): 102-3.

Chipman, Dawn. "Strike!" *Revolution: The Journal of Nursing Empowerment*, Winter 1993: 22-25, 81-83.

Christman, L. "Perspectives on Role Socialization of Nurses." *Nursing Outlook*, September/October 1991, 39(5): 209-12.

"CNA Files Consumer Fraud Lawsuit Against Alta Bates." *California Nurse*, October 1994, p. 9.

Cox, Helen. "Verbal Abuse Nationwide, Part II: Impact and Modifications." *Nursing Management*, March 1991, 22(3): 66-69.

Cunningham , Marilyn E., Chambers, Julie, Howard, Lee, and Schenk, Sharon. "The Student Management Team: A Vehicle for Empowerment." *Revolution: The Journal for Nursing Empowerment,* Spring 1994: 42-45.

Curran, Connie R., Minnick, Ann, Moss, Joan. "Who Needs Nurses?" *American Journal of Nursing*, April 1987, 87(4): 444-447.

Curtain, Leah. "Health Reform Proposals: Which is the Fairest of Them All?" *Nursing Management*, November 1993, 24(11): 7-8.

"Cutting RNs is a Risk." *The Business Journal*, May 30, 1994, p. 42.

Dean, Malcolm. "Nursing's Identity Crisis." *The Lancet*, May 9, 1992, (2): 1160.

Del Bueno, Dorothy J. "Power and Politics." *Nursing Outlook*, 34(3):124-128.

DeMoro, Rose Ann. "Most Frequently Asked Questions About the Effects of Restructuring." *California Nurse*, March 1995, p. 4.

"Denouncing Cuts, RN Groups Go Public with Safety Issues." *American Journal of Nursing*, April 1995, 95(4): 67, 71.

"Denver Nurses Go on Warpath to Get a Raise: Mass Walkout Threat Proves a Winning Strategy." *American Journal of Nursing*, August 1988, 88(8): 1132.

"Employers Get More Protection." *The Sacramento Bee*, June 1, 1994, p. F1.

"'ER Revives TV Hospital Dramatics; Nurses Rally to Make It Realistic." *American Journal of Nursing*, February 1995, 95(2): 77, 79.

Estela, Linda. *Alternative Careers in Nursing*, Hayward, CA: Nurses Research Publications, 1993.

Fassel, Gillian E. "A Courageous Voice for Nursing." *Nursing Outlook*, May/June 1991, 39(3): 115-119.

Fondiller, Shirley, RN, EdD. "Public Speaking: Try It—You'll Like It." *American Journal of Nursing*, March 1994, 94(3): 64-67.

__________. "Writing for Publication." *American Journal of Nursing*, August, 1994 94(8): 62-64.

Friedman, Emily. "Nursing: Breaking the Bonds?" *Journal of the American Medical Association*, Dec. 26, 1990, (5): 3117.

__________. "Nursing: New Power, Old Problems." *Journal of the American Medical Association*, Dec. 19, 1990, (4): 2977.

__________. "Troubled Past of an Invisible Profession." *Journal of the American Medical Association*, Dec. 12, 1990, (5): 2851.

Galen, Michele. "Cheaper Primary Care: Nurses May be the Answer." *Business Week*, April 12, 1993, (1): 71.

Gardner, Diane L., PhD, RN. "Issues Related to the Use of Nurse Extenders." *Journal of Nursing Administration*, October 1991, 21(10): 40-45.

Gasparis, Laura, RN, MA, CEN, CCRN, and Swirsky, Joan, RN, MS, CS. *Nurse Abuse*. New York: Power Press, 1993.

Genusa, Angela. "Perioperative RNs Face Changing Roles." *NURSEweek*, November 1994, 7(23): 1.

Gordon, Suzanne. "First Names Only." *Revolution: The Journal of Nursing Empowerment*, Fall 1993: 28-30, 102-103.

__________. "Healthcare Reform—How 'The System' Works Against Nurses." *Revolution: The Journal of Nursing Empowerment*, Fall 1993: 10-16, 97.

__________. "Nurses in the Canadian System: An Exclusive Interview with Alice Baumgart." *Revolution: The Journal of Nursing Empowerment*, Fall 1993: 18-22, 99.

__________. "R.N.s Beware! Healthcare 'Reform' May Give Your Job to a Tech!" *Revolution: The Journal of Nursing Empowerment*, Spring 1994: 14-17, 84-85.

__________. "Voices from the Frontlines—Nurses Speak Out!" *Revolution: The Journal of Nursing Empowerment*, Spring 1995: 24-30, 66.

Gordon, Suzanne and Baer, Ellen. "Cost-cutting is a Life-and-Death Issue as 'Nurse Substitutes' Roam Hospitals." *The Sacramento Bee*, December 7, 1994, p. B7.

Gorman, Christine. "Fed Up, Fearful and Frazzled; as a Profession Flounders, Patient Care Is Suffering," (Special Report: The Crisis in Nursing). *Time*, March 14, 1988, (2): 77.

Gorman, Sheila, and Clark, Noreen. "Power and Effective Nursing Practice." *Nursing Outlook*, May/June 1986, 34(3): 129-134.

Grandjean, Burke D., Aiken, Linda H., Bonjean, Charles M. "Professional Autonomy and the Work Satisfaction of Nursing Educators." *Nursing Research*, May/June 1976, 25 (3): 216-221.

Gray, Barbara B., MN, RN. "Nursing Organizations Regroup." *NURSEweek*, December 1994, 7(26): 1, 30.

__________. "RN says Nurses Must get Involved in Media." *NURSEweek*, February 1995 (first issue), p. 1, 20.

__________. "When RNs Face Violence and Abuse at Work." *NURSEweek*, January 4, 1993, p. 10-11.

Greenleaf, Nancy P. "The Politics of Self-Esteem." *Nursing Digest*, Fall 1978, p. 1-7.

Griffith, H. M. et al. "Nurses' Perspectives on a National Health Plan," *Nursing Outlook*, July/August 1991, 39(4): 178-82.

Hall, J. M. et al. "The Nursing Shortage in the Context of National Health Care." *Nursing Outlook*, March/April 1991, 39(2): 69-72.

"HCFA Report Cites Staffing Problems as Cause of Florida Hospital's Errors." *The American Nurse,* June 1995, p. 18.

"Health Care Field Continues to Beat Strong in Today's Job Ratings Chart." *The Sacramento Bee,* January 23, 1994, p. G8.

"Hearing on Alta Bates Fraud Suit Seen as Victory for RNs, Patients." *California Nurse,* March 1995, p. 3.

Himali, Ursula. "More Than 25,000 RNs March on Washington, Issuing a Wake-up Call to Consumers and Lawmakers." *The American Nurse,* April/May 1995, p. 1, 20-21.

Hodes, Jay R., and Van Crombrugghe, Phyllis. "Nurse-Physician Relationships." *Nursing Management,* July 1990, 21(7): 73-75.

Holcomb, Betty. "Nurses Fight Back." *Ms. Magazine,* June 1988, (7): 72.

"Illinois RNs Seek Compromise on Scope of Practice." *American Journal of Nursing,* January 1986, 86(1): 77.

"In Landmark Pact, Illinois RNs Win Staffing Guarantees." *American Journal of Nursing,* March 1995, (95)3: 67, 70-71.

Kalisch, Philip A., and Kalisch, Beatrice, J. "The Image of the Nurse in Motion Pictures." *American Journal of Nursing,* April 1982, (82)4: 605-611.

__________. "The Image of Nurses in Novels." *American Journal of Nursing,* August 1982, 82(8): 1220-1224.

__________. "Nursing Images: The TV News Picture." *Nursing Management,* April 1985, (16)4: 39-48.

Kelly, Lucie S. "Another Look at the Future of Health Care." *Nursing Outlook*, July/August 1991, 39(4): 150-151.

__________. "The Conundrum of Recycled Leadership." *Nursing Outlook*, January/February 1991, 39(1): 5.

Kelly, Lucie Young. "The Power of Powerlessness." *Nursing Outlook*, July 1978, 22(7): 468.

Ketter, Joni. "Employers Use Supreme Court Decision Against RNs; ANA Devises Legal, Legislative Strategies." *The American Nurse*, October 1994, 26(9): 1.

__________." Teamwork Ensured March's Success." *The American Nurse*, April/May 1995, p. 1, 21.

Kleiman, Carol. "Nurses Stand to Benefit from Health-Care Reform." *San Francisco Examiner*, March 20, 1994, p. 19.

Kusserow, Suzanne "The Guide to True Education—Life Experience." *Revolution: The Journal of Nursing Empowerment*, Summer 1994: 24-26.

Kutlenios, Rose M., and Bowman, Margaret H. "Oppression—How Nurses Can Overcome It." *Revolution: The Journal of Nursing Empowerment,* Summer 1994: 20-21, 100.

Kuzins, Rebecca. "Nurses Next in Line for Pain" *The Sacramento Business Journal*, May 30, 1994, p. 1.

Laskey, D. J. "The Power of Nursing" (letter). *American Journal of Nursing*, June 1992, 92(6): 25.

"Layoffs Loom as Kaiser Turns to 'Multiskilled Caregivers'." *American Journal of Nursing*, May 1994, 94(5): 77-82.

Leavitt, Judith Kline, RN, MEd, FAAN, and Mason, Diana J., RN, PhD, FAAN. "Finding Your Political Voice" *American Journal of Nursing*, October 1994, 94(10): 56.

Lecker, M. "Nursing's Image: A Factor in the Shortage" (letter). *Nursing Outlook*, May/June 1991, 39(3): 139.

Lee, Marietta. "AJN Interview: P.K. Scheerle." *American Journal of Nursing*, July 1994, 94(7): 38-40.

Lepler, Marcia. "Floating." *Revolution: The Journal of Nursing Empowerment*, Spring 1993: 10-18, 97.

Lewis, Joan D., et al. "Men in Nursing: Some Troubling Data." *American Journal of Nursing*, August 1990, 90(8): 30.

Liccardo, Lynn. "The Word on TV's Newest Nurses: Patience!" *Revolution: The Journal of Nursing Empowerment*, Spring 1995: 52-53.

Lippman, Doris Troth, RN, EdD, and Ponton, Karen Stonkas, RN, MA. "The Image of Nursing Among High School Guidance Counselors." *Nursing Outlook*, May/June 1993, 41(3): 129-134.

__________. "Nursing's Image on the University Campus." *Nursing Outlook*, January/February 1989, 37(1): 24-27.

Loeb, Susan J. "Wake Up Nurse Educators! Get with the Empowerment Program!" *Revolution: The Journal of Nursing Empowerment*, Winter 1993: 34-35, 85.

Maglacas, Amelia Mangay. "The Best Placed Profession." *World Health*, April 1988, (1): 25.

Manion, Jo, RN, MA, CNAA. "Nurse Intrapreneurs: The Heroes of Health Care's Future." *Nursing Outlook*, January/February 1991, 39(1): 18-21.

__________. "The Nurse Intrapreneur: How to Motivate from Within." *American Journal of Nursing*, January 1994, 94(1): 38-42.

Martin, E. Jane, White, Joyce E., Hansen, Marie M. "Preparing Students to Shape Health Policy." *Nursing Outlook*, March/April 1989, 37 (2): 89-93.

Mason, Diana J., Backer, Barbara A., and Georges, C. Alicia. "Toward a Feminist Model for the Political Empowerment of Nurses," *Revolution: The Journal of Nursing Empowerment,* Spring 1993: 62-71, 106-107.

McKee, Bradford A. "From Bedside to Business." *Nation's Business*, Jan. 1990, (1): 50.

McKibbin, Richard C. The Nursing Shortage and the 1990's: Realities and Remedies. Kansas City: American Nurses Association, 1990.

McVeigh, D. et al. "Career Mobility for RNs." *Nursing Outlook*, January/February 1991, 39(1): 30-1.

"The 'Media Model' Theory of Nursing." *Nursing Forum*, January-March 1992, 27(1):35- 36.

"Men in Nursing" (letters, comment). *American Journal of Nursing*, November 1990, 90(11): 27.

Meyer, C. "Nursing on the Political Front." *American Journal of Nursing*, Oct. 1992, (10): 56-60, 63-4.

Mikulencak, Mandy "Fact or Fiction? Nursing and Realism on TV's Newest Medical Drama. *The American Nurse*, March 1995, p. 31.

"Minnesota's Healthcare Reform Law Sets New Standard for Other States; RNs Were

Leaders in Reform Push." *American Journal of Nursing*, June 1992, 92(6): 80.

"Missouri NPs Win Appeal in Medical Practice Suit." *American Journal of Nursing*, January 1984, 84(1): 111.

"More on Men in Nursing" (letters, comments). *American Journal of Nursing*, February 1991, 91(2): 24.

Murphy, N. J. "Nursing Leadership in Health Policy Decision Making." *Nursing Outlook*, July/August 1992, 40(4): 158-61.

Murphy, Suzanne Z. "Don't be a Doormat: Personal Empowerment in Nursing." *Revolution: The Journal of Nursing Empowerment*, Summer 1994: 66-68.

National Nurses in Business Association. *How I Became a Nurse Entrepreneur: Tales from 50 Nurses in Business.* Petaluma, CA: National Nurses in Business Association, 1991.

"Nation's RNs Stand Up to be Counted in Reform Fight." *American Journal of Nursing*, May 1994, 94(5): 79-81.

Nawrocki, Helene, RN. The Nurses Book of Courage. Newton, PA: Center for Nursing Excellence, 1993.

"New Salary Battle Pits Maine vs. Massachusetts Hospitals." *American Journal of Nursing*, August 1988, 88(8): 1133.

"The Newest Layoff Strategy: Forcing Nurses to Compete to Keep Their Jobs" *American Journal of Nursing*, November 1993, 93(11): 86.

"NLN Members Back Graduate Nursing Preparation for Advanced Practice." *American Journal of Nursing*, November 1993, 93(11): 75.

"Nurses, Administration Encouraged to Work Together in Cutting Costs." *NURSEweek*, February 1995, 8(3): 2.

"Nurses Are Ready to Fight the AMA for a Wider Role." *The Sacramento Bee*, March 28, 1994, p. C3.

"Nurses Win Battle for a Research Center at NIH; Congress Rebukes Reagan and Overrides His Veto." *American Journal of Nursing*, January 1986, 86(1): 75.

"Nursing Administration Can Enhance the Image of the Nurse." *Journal of Nursing Administration*, September 1991, 21(9): 7-8.

"Nursing: Rewards vs. Frustrations." *USA Today*, October 1990, p. 10.

"Nursing: Who's to Blame for Poor Image?" *USA Today*, October 1989, p. 10-11.

Oder, Norman. "Memoirs Issued from The Medical Front." *Publishers Weekly*, February 24, 1995, p. 31.

Palmer, P. N. "Nurses Must be Visible in Health Care Reform as Well as in its Delivery" (editorial). *AORN Journal*, February 1992, 55(2): 451-2.

Palmer, P. N. "Physician Bonding: An Insult to Both Physicians and Nurses" (editorial). *AORN Journal*, May 1992, 55(5): 1159-60.

Parks, John E., RN. "Men in Nursing" (letters). *American Journal of Nursing*, November 1990, 90(11): 27.

Paternostro, J. M. "Nursing Administrators Can Enhance the Image of the Nurse." *Journal of Nursing Administration*, September 1991, 21(9): 7-8.

Pender, N. J. "Health Care Reform: One View of the Future." *Nursing Outlook*, March/April 1993, 41(2): 56-7.

Perry, Sarah J. "Thoughts on the Nursing Power Shortage." *Revolution: The Journal of Nursing Empowerment*, Spring 1993: 58-60.

Pillitteri, A. et al. "'Doctor-Nurse' Game: a Comparison of 100 years—1888-1990" *Nursing Outlook*, May/June 1993, 41(3): 113-6.

Porter-O'Grady, Tim, RN, CS, EdD. "Working with Consultants on a Redesign." *American Journal of Nursing*, October 1994, 94(10): 33-37.

Pulitzer, Lisa Beth. "Short Staffed and Working Scared—Can Nurses Just Say 'No'?" *Revolution: The Journal of Nursing Empowerment*, Summer 1993: 10-13, 98-102.

Quirolo, Lynn, RN. "ANA Hears Staff Nurse Perspective on Restructuring." *California Nurse*, March 1995, p. 2.

Resnick, Susan K. "Twentysomething Nurses." *Revolution: The Journal of Nursing Empowerment*, Summer 1993: 18-26.

"Rewards vs. Frustration." *USA Today*, Oct. 1990, (1): 10.

Reynolds, Gloria Jean. "Hospitals—Our Patriarchal Institutions." *Revolution: The Journal of Nursing Empowerment*, Spring 1995: 58-62.

"RNs Aim to Mend Gap in Clinton Plan; AMA Attacks Advanced Practice Roles." *American Journal of Nursing*, January 1994, 94(1): 83-89.

"RNs, Patients Describe Care Crisis to Senate Committee" *California Nurse,* March 1995, p.3.

"RN Population Grows to 2.2 Million; Nurses Age a Bit but Work More." *American Journal of Nursing*, October 1994, 94(10): 68.

Roberts, Susan Jo. "Feminism & Nursing: Oppressed Group Behavior—Implications for Nursing" *Revolution: The Journal for Nursing Empowerment*, Fall 1994: 28-34.

Rochford, Kate. "Nurses United Can Create Change." *Revolution: The Journal of Nursing Empowerment*, Summer 1994: 60-62, 109.

Roedel, Rita R., and Nystrom, Paul C. "Nursing Jobs and Satisfaction." *Nursing Management*, February 1988, 19(2): 34-38.

Schmidt, Bob. "Within the Capitol Nurses Fight Against Hospitals and Physicians." *The Business Journal*, November 1, 1993, p. 16.

Schoen, Delores C., RN, PhD. "Nurses Attitudes Toward Control Over Nursing Practice." *Nursing Forum*, January-March 1992, 27(1): 27-34.

Schlomann, Pamela. "Burnout or Exploitation?" *Revolution: The Journal of Nursing Empowerment*, Winter 1993: 20-21.

Schorr, Thelma M., RN. "Nurse-Run Managed Care?" *American Journal of Nursing*, October 1990, 90(10): 25.

__________. "Will Nurses Contract Their Services?" *American Journal of Nursing*, October 1990, 90(10): 39.

Seago, Jean Ann. "Verbal Abuse of Nurses." *Revolution: The Journal of Nursing Empowerment*, Fall 1993: 62-64, 106.

Spitzer, Roxanne B., RN, MA, and Davivier, Maryann PhD. "Nursing in the 1990's: Expanding Opportunities." *Nursing Administration Quarterly*, Winter 1987, 11(2): 55-61.

Stearley, Harold. "Battered But Not Beaten—The Politics of Victimization" *Revolution: The Journal of Nursing Empowerment*, Spring 1995: 63-64.

__________. "Defensive Nursing." *Revolution: The Journal of Nursing Empowerment*, Fall 1994: 43-45.

__________. "Professional Jealousy—The No-Win Factor." *Revolution: The Journal of Nursing Empowerment*, Winter, 1994: 52-53.

__________. "Restructuring and the A.N.A.—Whose Side Are They On?" *Revolution: The Journal of Nursing Empowerment*, Fall 1994: 36-42.

Stein, Leonard I., Watts, David T., and Howell, Timothy. "The Doctor-Nurse Game Revisited," *Nursing Outlook*, November/December 1990, 38(6): 264-268.

Stocker, S. "Unravelling the Leadership Conundrum." *Nursing Outlook*, July/August 1991, 39(4): 188-9.

"Striking New York Nurses 'Fast for Justice'." *American Journal of Nursing*, March 1995, 95(3): 67.

Summers, Caryn, RN. *Caregiver, Caretaker.* Salt Lake City, UT: Commune-a-key Publishing, 1992.

Swirsky, Joan. "Exclusive *Revolution* Interview with Virginia Trotter Betts, President of the American Nurses Association." *Revolution: The Journal of Nursing Empowerment,* Spring 1993: 40-48.

"Title 22 Hearings: RNs Urge DHS to Protect Patients" *California Nurse,* March 1995, p. 7.

"Top Ten Myths About Hospital Restructuring and Healthcare Reform." *Revolution: The Journal for Nursing Empowerment,* Fall 1994: 24-25.

Weisfeld, N. E., et al. "Toward a National Policy for Nursing." *Nursing Outlook,* March/April 1991, 39(2): 73-76.

"Who's to Blame for Poor Image?" *USA Today,* Oct. 1989, (2): 10.

Will, George F. "The Dignity of Nursing: The American Ideal of a Doctor—Kindly, Caring, Reassuring Dr. Welby—Was Essentially a Nurse." Newsweek, May 23, 1988, (1): 80.

"Will Information Technology Solve the Shortage?" *American Journal of Nursing,* October 1990, 90(10): 41.

Wolf, Gail A. "Nursing Turnover: Some Causes and Solutions." *Nursing Outlook,* April 1981, 29(4): 233-236.

Wooten, Patty, RN, Editor. *Heart Humor & Healing,* Salt Lake City, UT: Commune-a-key Publishing, 1994.

Index

A

B

C

D

E

F

G

H

I

J

K

L

M

N

O

P

R

S

T

U

W

About The Author

Jane Schweitzer was born and raised in San Francisco, California. She graduated from the two-year nursing program offered by City College of San Francisco in 1966, then worked as an operating room nurse in various hospitals throughout California for more than fifteen years. In addition, Ms. Schweitzer has several years of experience as a journalist and free lance writer.

The author completed her undergraduate studies at the University of California, Berkeley where she earned a B.A. in Russian History in 1982. Graduate studies at the University of San Francisco resulted in a Masters in Public Administration.

Ms. Schweitzer lives in Fair Oaks, California, with her husband, author/publisher Alan Canton, four cats, and an Australian Shepherd.